Advance Praise for
"What Every Man Really Needs!"
By Ira Epstein

"This is a great book. I've already lost 7 pounds
from Ira's advice. Every man should read it!"
-Jim Miller, Port Jefferson, New York

"My husband needs to read this book. Ira tells it like it is."
- "This book can help make all men better husbands."
-Amy Esposito, Commack, New York

"All I have to do is eat better and have more sex? "
I love this book!"
-Michael Sudyn, Manhattan, New York

"Ira's written a great book that deals with every aspect
of my life that I would like to make better".
-Edward Epstein, Manchester, Connecticut

WHAT EVERY MAN
REALLY NEEDS!

(The men's guide to better eating and more sex)
By Ira Epstein

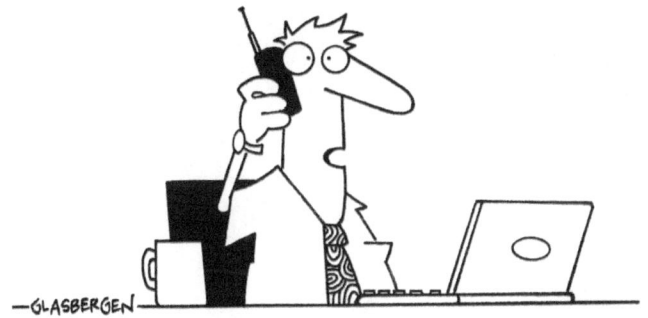

"How can you say I'm not romantic? Yesterday I almost
thought about maybe buying you some flowers!"

The First Real Healthy Living Plan for Men

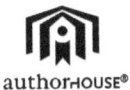

authorHOUSE®

AuthorHouse™
1663 Liberty Drive
Bloomington, IN 47403
www.authorhouse.com
Phone: 1-800-839-8640

This book is intended as a reference volume only. The information given here is designed to help you make informed decisions about your health. It is not intended as a substitute for any treatment that may have been prescribed by your doctor. If you suspect that you have a medical problem, I urge you to seek competent medical help.

First published by AuthorHouse 07/27/2011

ISBN: 978-1-4634-2673-6 (sc)
ISBN: 978-1-4634-2672-9 (hc)
ISBN: 978-1-4634-2671-2 (ebk)

Library of Congress Control Number: 2011911273

Printed in the United States of America

Any people depicted in stock imagery provided by Thinkstock are models, and such images are being used for illustrative purposes only.
Certain stock imagery © Thinkstock.

This book is printed on acid-free paper.

Because of the dynamic nature of the Internet, any web addresses or links contained in this book may have changed since publication and may no longer be valid. The views expressed in this work are solely those of the author and do not necessarily reflect the views of the publisher, and the publisher hereby disclaims any responsibility for them.

To Melinda, my wife and partner in life, whose love and encouragement helped me to become a better man

TABLE OF CONTENTS

Part 2 – Exercise Can Be Fun and Rewarding

INTRODUCTION

Why a "healthy living" plan for men?

It's a fact that most men do not eat or exercise properly and stop paying attention to the relationship with their partners. This can cause a multitude of health related problems and eventually will affect their relationships and that will affect how often they get to have sex.

There are so many diet books and programs out there. And almost all of these diet plans are targeted at women, even though both men and women use them. There are reasons for this.

1. Women diet to feel good about
2. themselves.
3. Women worry about what others think of
4. them and respond to this pressure.
5. Women will try any fad diet to lose weight
6. quickly.

Men, on the other hand, do not diet. They only want to lose weight if and when it becomes a problem for them physically or medically. Men believe they are never going to die or get seriously ill, so in their minds, what is the point.

The major problem with diets is that they all cater to the idea that losing weight quickly is a worthwhile goal. The majority of these *fad diets* are just re-creations of older diets that have failed. These diets are also built around women's physiology and completely ignore the specific nutritional needs of men. The American Medical Association and The American Dieticians Association both agree that in the long run these diets are unhealthy and could lead to serious health problems, especially for men.

The other problem is lack of exercise. Men need to exercise to maintain their bone and muscle mass and to burn unwanted calories.

One of the best exercises for men is sex. The health benefits are many, and it is something men will do any time the opportunity is presented.

It is said that, *"a women can use sex to get what she wants, but a man can't because sex is what he wants!"* And in order for men to be able to have a greater intimate relationship and reap the health benefits from a more active sex life, they must learn how to communicate better with their significant others.

How does this book relate to men and their health?

This book will educate and illuminate men on how to change their lifestyle to a healthy one. As a result, they will not only lose weight but they will also get the exercise they need and increase their enjoyment of life's pleasures: primarily, a better sexual relationship with their significant others.

I want to specifically thank Dr. Clay Tucker-Ladd (1931-2010) for his help and support on the sections in my book on relationship building and stress reduction.

CHAPTER 1 - WHY DO WE EAT AND WHY DIET?

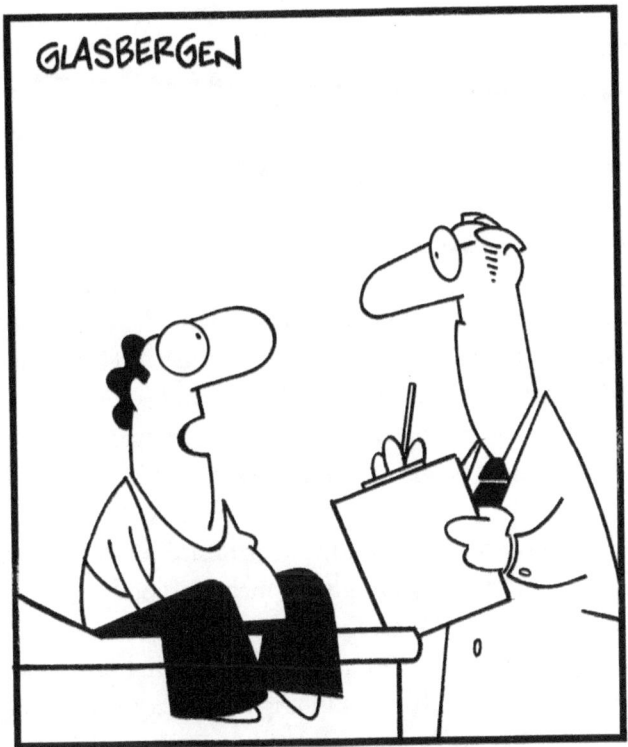

GLASBERGEN

"Eat less and exercise more? That's the
most ridiculous fad diet I've heard of yet!"

Why do we eat?

We basically do not eat because we are hungry. Hunger is when
the body needs food to provide energy in order to perform the basic
metabolic tasks, such as breathing and pumping blood, and extra tasks
such as working and playing. Many people eat because it's the time
of day (breakfast, lunch and dinner time) or as a result of depression,
boredom or habit (like when you are watching TV).

How much you eat isn't just a matter of willpower or the lack of it.
It is a biological process that drives our ability to survive. Trying to lose

1

weight by using diets and food restrictions is counterproductive and only causes the body to trigger chemical reactions to stimulate your appetite and increase your hunger. This creates a vicious cycle of over-eating because of a complex system of chemical and hormonal reactions that tell you to eat.

How hunger works

The hypothalamus is partly responsible for processing eating behavior. The cells in the hypothalamus communicate with cells in other parts of the brain to coordinate the release of chemicals that form the feedback system that helps regulate how much and what you eat.

When the body needs nourishment, neurotransmitters (chemicals that transmit information to the neurons or brain cells) are released. Current research is being done to help explain the exact mechanism, but one neurotransmitter called Neuropeptide Y (NPY) is thought to respond when the body needs carbohydrates. According to the theory, low levels of glycogen (carbohydrate in storage form in your body) and low blood sugar levels stimulate NPY's release from the hypothalamus.

As NPY levels increase, so does your desire for sweet and starchy foods. While you sleep, your glycogen and blood sugar stores are used up, and they send a message to the brain to release NPY. It's no coincidence that our favorite morning foods are rich in carbohydrates-cereal, breads, bagels, and fruit. Skipping breakfast increases NPY levels so that by afternoon you need a carbohydrate binge. This craving for carbs is an innate biological urge at work, not a lack of willpower. Stress and dieting are thought to trigger NPY production as well.

Eating carbohydrates or other favorite foods turn off NPY by using a serotonin feedback system. Serotonin is another neurotransmitter that is associated with the feeling of fullness and satisfaction. When serotonin increases, NPY decreases, telling your body that you have had enough food and you can stop eating.

Another neurotransmitter called galanin is released when the fat stores need replenishment. Research on galanin has been conducted only on animals, but the human appetite for fat is believed to act in a similar way. Laboratory animals that have been injected with galanin prefer high-fat foods to high-carbohydrate ones. And when animals were given drugs that interfered with the galanin production, their preference for fat decreased. How galanin works may help explain why some people store more fat than others do. In the evening, galanin levels tend to rise, which may be the body's way of making sure that people have enough calories to last them through the night without taking in more food.

Motivation

Long-term weight loss is a matter of attitude and conditioning. What the short-time diets focus on is "the don'ts", denial, and immediate results, without allowing room for slip-ups. You need to focus on making healthier choices, enjoy feeling better, be healthier and more energized, establish flexible, short- term attainable goals and leave room for indulgences. When you feel good about yourself, you have more energy and want to continue eating better and feeling healthier.

To accomplish this, you need to emphasize healthy eating and exercise.

Why diet at all?

Your degree of risk for developing weight-related health problems depends not only on how overweight you are, but also where you store the excess fat. Body fat that accumulates around the stomach area poses a greater health risk than fat stored in the lower body. Typically, men are prone to building up fat in the stomach area, developing a "beer belly" or "pot belly". Men are more apt to develop diabetes, high blood pressure, heart disease, and certain types of cancer with this condition. Reducing your weight by only 5 to 10 percent increases your HDL levels (the good cholesterol) while reducing LDL and triglyceride levels, which are associated with increased risk of heart disease.

CHAPTER 2 - WHY FAD DIETS DON'T WORK

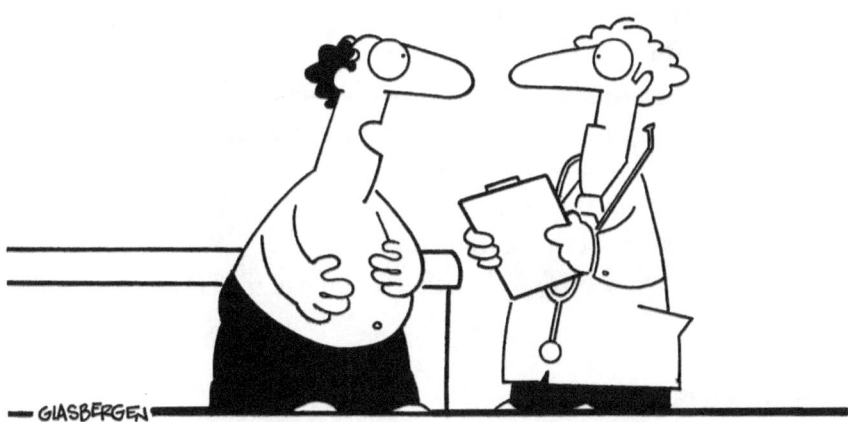

"I'm dieting faithfully. For breakfast I follow the Egg Lovers Diet. At lunch, I switch to the Fast Food Diet. For dinner, I do the Steak-n-Pasta Diet. And during TV I switch to the Chip-n-Dip Diet."

This chapter explains and exposes some of the different popular fad diets that all promise the same thing: Quick and easy weight loss. As men, we are naturally skeptical about the "new and revolutionary" diet plans that are simply rehashes of old programs that use current scientific weight-loss vocabulary and a little technical- sounding mumbo jumbo to sell us on diets that will fail. These "doctors and self styled nutritionists" count on the public's lack of knowledge about nutrition to bamboozle millions of dollars out of our pockets. The women buy into this because they will try anything to look like the fashion models or movie stars who have figures that are not the norm.

The key to successful weight loss is not rocket science. What all these fad diets don't tell you is that your body will lose weight if you do two things; reduce your calories and exercise. When you go on one of these fad diets you will lose weight quickly because the body's metabolism thinks you are starving and will burn its stored fat. But then your metabolism will slow down to conserve the energy stored and you will stop losing weight. This results in frustration and causes you to go off the diet, and over-eat, and gain back the weight you lost (and sometimes more). You then try another fad diet and the cycle repeats itself. This yo-yo effect is detrimental to your health.

High-protein, low carbohydrate diets have been widely promoted in recent years as an effective approach to losing weight. These diets generally recommend that dieters receive 30% to 50% of their total calories from protein. By comparison, the American Heart Association, the National Cholesterol Education Program and the American Cancer Society all recommend a diet in which only 10% to 15% of calories are derived from protein (nutrients essential to the building, maintenance and repair of tissues in the body).

The following is a brief explanation of some of the fad diets currently out there:

The Atkins Diet:

The Premise

By restricting carbohydrates drastically to a mere fraction of that found in the typical American diet, the body goes into a different metabolic state called *ketosis*, whereby it burns its own fat for fuel. Normally the body burns carbohydrates for fuel -- this is the main source of fuel for your brain, heart and many other organs. A person in ketosis is getting energy from *ketones*, little carbon fragments that are the fuel created by the breakdown of fat stores. When the body is in ketosis, you tend to feel less hungry, and thus you're likely to eat less than you might otherwise. As a result, your body changes from a carbohydrate-burning engine into a fat-burning engine. So instead of relying on the carbohydrate-rich items you might typically consume for energy, and leaving your fat stores just where they were before (the hips, belly, and thighs), your fat stores become a primary energy source. The purported result is weight loss.

The Reality:

In diets that contain fewer than 900 calories, all food eaten (including protein and fat) is broken down into glucose to provide fuel for the body. Protein and fat are very expensive fuels for your body. You can only convert 70 percent of the protein and 30 percent of the fat you eat to glucose. The nitrogen from the protein is excreted in the urine. This leaves no protein for repair or maintenance of muscles and organs. Also, in diets containing fewer than 130 grams of carbohydrates, ketosis occurs and your body starts breaking down muscle and lean tissue to provide glucose for brain and nerve fuel. Your body's first need is for fuel. Your body's use of dietary fuels cannot be changed drastically by altering your diet.

Your body can and does take stored fat (as triglycerides) and incompletely breaks it down into ketones, which can be used as a fuel source for muscles and organs. To completely break down body fat, you need glucose and oxygen. If glucose is not available for fuel by your limiting dietary carbohydrates, your body learns to run on ketones. However your brain doesn't. Your brain gets sluggish because it only runs on glucose. Your body starts breaking down muscle and organ tissue to provide the needed glucose for brain tissue. Protein contains glucose in its structure and it can be scavenged for use by the brain and nerves.

Quick weight loss diets claim they spare muscle protein, but they don't. A diet high in protein and low in carbohydrates does not spare muscle protein from being broken down, unless you eat enough carbohydrate. As you continue on a high protein, low carbohydrate diet, the amount of ketones increases and ketosis occurs. Ketones are very irritating to your kidneys and the kidneys try to get rid of the ketones through the urine.

High protein diets can cause a number of health problems, including:

Kidney failure- Consuming too much protein puts a strain on the kidneys, which can make a person susceptible to kidney disease.

High cholesterol- It is well known that high protein diets (consisting of red meat, whole dairy products, and other high fat foods) are linked to high cholesterol. Studies have linked high cholesterol levels to an increased risk of developing heart disease and cancer.

Osteoporosis and kidney stones- High-protein diets have also been shown to cause people to excrete more calcium than normal through their urine. Over a prolonged period of time, this can increase a person's risk of osteoporosis and kidney stones.

Cancer- One of the reasons high protein diets increase the risks of certain health problems is the avoidance of carbohydrate- containing foods and the vitamins, minerals, fiber and anti-oxidants they contain. It is therefore important to obtain your protein from a diet rich in whole grains, fruits and vegetables. Not only are your needs for protein being met, but you are also helping to reduce your risk of developing cancer.

Unhealthy metabolic state (ketosis) - Low carb diets can cause your body to go into a dangerous metabolic state called ketosis since your body burns fat instead of glucose for energy. During ketosis, the body forms substances known as *ketones*, which can cause organs to fail and result in gout, kidney stones, or kidney failure. Ketones can also dull a person's appetite, cause nausea and bad breath. Eating at least 100 grams of carbohydrates a day prevents ketosis.

The South Beach Diet:

The Premise:

Miami cardiologist Dr. Arthur Agatston invented this diet in order to help his cardiac patients maintain a healthy lifestyle and lose weight.

The idea behind the diet involves carbohydrates. The aim of the South Beach Diet is to clear your diet of the types of carbohydrates and fats that can lead to weight gain. The diet distinguishes "good" carbohydrates from "bad" carbohydrates, and purports that by cutting the bad carbs out of your diet you will lower your body's levels of cholesterol and insulin which will ultimately lead to weight loss.

The diet is actually based on the idea that high-glycemic carbohydrates (those that rate higher than 55 on the glycemic scale), or "bad" carbohydrates, such as white bread and white rice, lead to weight gain. The South Beach Diet thus recommends that dieters consume more low-glycemic carbohydrates or "good" carbohydrates such as whole grains and vegetables, which take longer to break down, expend more energy as they break down, and don't lead to empty cravings.

The South Beach Diet claims that most people who follow the diet will lose 8 to 13 pounds after the first two weeks (although it is not certain whether this weight loss is actually the loss of fat or water). Then, if the basic rules of the diet are adhered to during Phases 2 and 3, you should be able to maintain your desired weight.

The diet should also help lower your blood cholesterol level, since it restricts the consumption of saturated fats. The diet should also discourage your body from storing the carbohydrates that you eat as fats, since you are instructed to eat mainly complex carbohydrates that take longer to break down than simple carbohydrates do.

The Reality:

These theories of weight loss remain unproven, and most experts are concerned that high-protein, low carb diets can cause a host of problems, particularly for the large segment of the population that is at risk for heart disease. What's more, the plan doesn't permit a high intake of fruits and vegetables, recommended by most nutrition experts because of the numerous documented health benefits from these foods.

The experts say that to achieve permanent weight loss you must change your lifestyle. This means following a lower calorie diet that includes grains, legumes, fruits and vegetables combined with participating in regular physical activity.

The Pritikin Principle:

The Premise:

Everyone who's ever thought about going on a diet has at least heard of The Pritikin Approach: a low-fat diet, not vegetarian, but largely based on vegetables, grains and fruits. Fat in the diet accounts for a mere 10%. Since 1976, more than 70,000 people have spent time at the Pritikin Longevity Centers learning how to eat healthy, prepare low-fat meals and snacks, and incorporate exercise and stress-reduction techniques into their lives. Several books by Nathan Pritikin carried the message of the Pritikin approach to the masses. It was an approach designed largely to promote well being by lowering cholesterol and helping diabetics normalize their blood sugar without taking insulin. That people lost weight was an added plus.

Now his son Robert has taken over and tweaked the concept. The same plant-based foods of the original are the staples of his diet, and the fat content of the regimen is still about as low as you can go.

But Robert's latest book, *The Pritikin Principle* (following *The New Pritikin Program* and *The Pritikin Weight Loss Breakthrough*), focuses on something he calls "The Calorie Density Solution".

He claims the concern is not calories but rather how dense they are in any given food. Fill up on foods that have relatively few calories per pound and you will lose the "excess body fat that threatens your health and longevity."

Choosing foods that are not "calorie-dense," such as apples and oatmeal, promises to "give you the freedom to eat until you are full and never limit your portions or be hungry in order to lose weight." The higher the caloric density of any given food, the more likely it is to cause weight gain because you will consume more calories to feel full than if you choose foods with a lower caloric density. A pound of broccoli, for instance, has only 130 calories (that's raw and unbuttered, of course), but a pound of chocolate chip cookies has 2,140 calories. You get the drift -- broccoli, good; chocolate chip cookies, bad.

The Reality:

Both the Pritikin diet and the nutritionally similar Ornish diet are extremely low in fat, Hill notes, down to 10% of total calories. "Yes, if we could do that we would all be healthier, but it is very hard to follow that formula in our environment," he cautions. "It's difficult to maintain such a low-fat content of our diets if you eat out often, and it takes time to prepare good tasting, low-fat food. Most people do not have the time to spend hours each day preparing food."

There seems to be little dispute that you will lose weight on the Pritikin diet or that it is generally a nutritionally rich diet low in calories. But there are warnings: "Because fat makes one feel full, the extremely low fat content of this diet will make those following it often feel hungry," says Teryl L. Tanaka, RD, the clinical nutrition manager at the Santa Monica UCLA Medical Center. Consequently, she adds, the likelihood is high of the weight returning after one stops strictly adhering to the diet.

"Another problem," says Tanaka, is that the low-fat content may actually be harmful to our health. "Pritikin also inhibits the intake and absorption of fat-soluble vitamins, and can even limit the amount of essential fatty acids provided by the diet needed for normal cell function, healthy skin and tissue, growth and development."

What do most nutritionists and health authorities like about the diet? Its strict limit of animal products -- often associated with a variety of major diseases -- and that it incorporates exercise and stress reduction, along with overall low calorie intake. But this is qualified with a concern that the extremely low-fat regimen is difficult to stick with over the long haul.

The Grapefruit Diet

The Premise:

So what is the *grapefruit diet* all about? The grapefruit diet promises that you can lose up to 50 pounds in as little as two and a half months time. Are you kidding? Not only is this type of weight loss very unhealthy, but is also nearly impossible without totally depriving your body of nutrients. The grapefruit diet consists of eating four meals throughout each day. Meal 1 would consist of a half *grapefruit,* 3 eggs (any style), and two slices of bacon! Healthy? I don't think so. Meal 2 would consist of another half grapefruit, any piece of meat you want, and a salad with any type of dressing. Is salad dressing healthy? No. Meal 3 consists of the exact same thing as meal 2, but add 1 cup of coffee into your meal. Finally, Meal 4 consists of either 1 eight-ounce glass of tomato juice or 1 eight-ounce glass of skim milk.

The Reality:

This is one of those diets that many of you may have tried in the past and found that it didn't work. Although the *grapefruit diet* seems very easy, it doesn't produce results and is far from a healthy and permanent way of dieting.

The Zone diet:

The Premise:

What is *The Zone*? Besides being the title of a mega-seller diet book, the Zone is a place where we find ourselves "feeling alert, refreshed, and full of energy," according to author Barry Sears, Ph.D. Sears, a former researcher in bio technology at the Massachusetts Institute of Technology, and the book's co-author Bill Lawren maintain that life in the Zone is what wellness is all about.

Like other popular diet books, *The Zone* offers more than just weight-loss claims. By retooling your metabolism with a diet that is 30% protein, 30% fat, and 40% carbohydrates, The Zone contends that you can expect to turn back encroaching heart disease, high blood pressure, and diabetes. Another much-touted advantage is better athletic performance. Sears doesn't come right out and claim he has found the cure for heart disease or diabetes, or how to win athletic competitions, but instead he provides glowing anecdotes from people who have taken *The Zone* to heart.

What *The Zone* does boldly claim is that much of the current thinking about good nutrition -- a diet high in carbohydrates, low in protein, and fats -- is "dead wrong". What's more, Sears contends, that type of diet has contributed to our risk of contracting serious, even life-threatening ailments such as heart disease, diabetes, and possibly cancer.

As a former scientist, Sears devotes considerable time to discussion of the science on which he based his theory. Simply stated, the Zone is a "metabolic state in which the body works at peak efficiency," and that state is created by eating a set ratio of carbohydrates, protein, and fat.

The Reality:

The Zone's eating plan is a combination of a small amount of low-fat protein at every meal, fats, and carbohydrates in the form of fiber-rich vegetables and fruits. The plan establishes a ratio for which Sears contends the body is genetically programmed (that 40-30-30 figure). And yes, we'll be thinner to boot.

Sears claims that the diet is based on his 15 years of research in bio nutrition. Although the book is full of success stories, including those of elite athletes, research that validates his specific claims isn't there. That doesn't mean that Sears' theories are wrong; it's just that no scientific evidence has proven that his program works.

Sears bases his theory on using diet to control the body's production of the hormone insulin. Among insulin's many roles, it helps regulate storage of excess energy as fat. The goal is to keep a balance between fat-storing insulin and the hormone glucagon, insulin's opposite, whose job it is to release the stored glucose from the liver when it is needed. Maintaining the correct balance between the two is accomplished by watching the size and specific content of your meals. In other words, you must be mindful of what you put on your plate. Sears suggests that we think of food not as "a source of calories but as a control system for hormones."

The Zone draws mixed reviews from nutrition experts. Researchers at the Center for Science in the Public Interest, which rated several fad diets, recently put it on their acceptable list, unlike Dr. Atkins *New Diet Revolution, Sugar Busters, The Carbohydrate Addict's Diet*, and *Protein Power*. "If you ignore the scientific rhetoric, the diet isn't bad," says Bonnie Liebman, MS, nutrition director for the center's publication, *Nutrition Action Healthletter*. As a caveat, she points out that the diet restricts carbohydrates more than necessary. "You are getting carbohydrates from fruit and vegetables on the diet, but a lot of the science is bunk," she says. What she likes is that the diet is relatively easy to follow: "You have a piece of protein the size of your palm, and you fill the rest of your plate up with fruits and vegetables."

Susan Roberts, Ph.D., head of the Weight Regulation Program at Tufts University and a professor of medicine and psychiatry there, also gives *The Zone* a qualified thumbs up. "Like most fad diet books, *The Zone* takes one of the several known controllers of energy, blood glucose, and blows it up into a whole book," she says. "It downplays the other factors that also determine how hungry we get and how much we eat, such as fiber and the caloric density of the food."

Roberts also finds fault with some of *The Zone's* food recommendations, such as that high-fat ice cream. Sears says it's OK because it won't raise your blood sugar precipitously, but it's not OK for other reasons, Roberts notes. To begin with, the cream in the ice cream is saturated fat, which isn't good for your overall cholesterol. (To be fair to the diet, Sears only allows a half-cup and certainly doesn't suggest you make it a habit.) Other nutritional experts, including some of Sears' former colleagues, are critical of his conclusions from the scientific evidence, contending that he has distorted or exaggerated the meaning of much of the basic research. They point out that no direct studies to verify his conclusions have been performed

The nutritional needs that are overlooked

The dangerous long-term effects of these diets when they are stringently followed are that they restrict your intake of the necessary vitamins and nutrients that your body needs.

One example is zinc. Zinc is perhaps the most important nutrient for a man's sexuality. Zinc is crucial for the production of sperm and seminal fluid. Zinc reduces the pituitary's production of *prolactin*, a hormone that inhibits the production of testosterone, without which a man's sexual libido decreases. Wheat germ, beans, red meat, crab and oysters are all high zinc-containing foods. Oysters have the most zinc concentrations and vitamin B12, which is one of the reasons, that oysters is considered to be an aphrodisiac. Further examples are explained in chapter 4.

Successful weight loss means you keep it off, some researchers say for at least one year after you have reached your proper weight range. Why not keep the weight off for the rest of your life? Research has proven that successful weight loss is accomplished through a slow weight loss process using a moderate calorie reduction, 30 minutes of exercise 4-5 times per week, and just watching what you eat.

The experts say that in order to achieve permanent weight loss you must change your lifestyle. This means following a lower calorie diet that includes whole grains, legumes, fruits and vegetables combined with participating in regular physical activity.

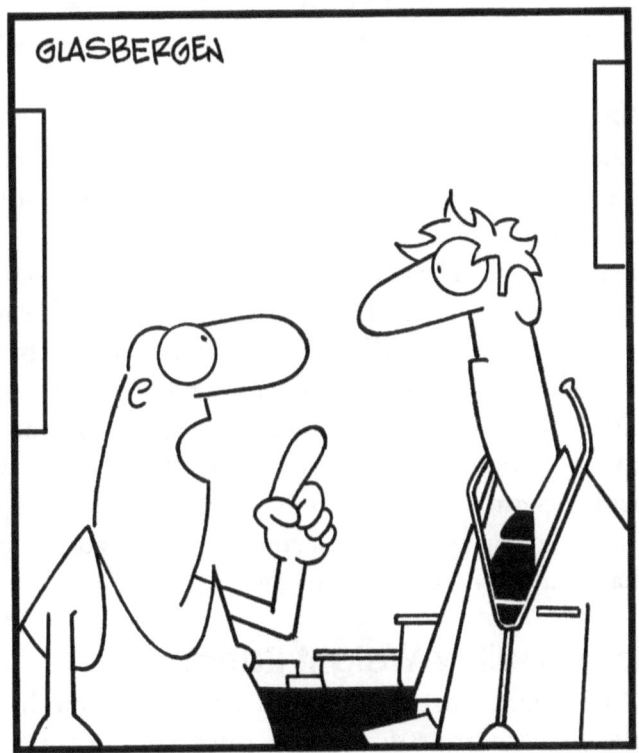

**"Dinosaurs didn't smoke cigarettes,
drink alcohol, or eat junk food...
*and where are they now!?"***

Your age affects your weight:

According to studies published in *The American Journal of Clinical Nutrition 53, 1991*, and *The Archives of Internal Medicine 150, 1990*, men gain an average of 10 pounds starting at age 25 and stabilize at about age 45. They begin to lose weight at about age 55. For both men and women, weight gain is highest in people aged 25 to 34 years.

Calorie needs peak at about age 25 and then begins to decline by about 2 percent every 10 years. So, if you're 25 years old and need 2,200 calories to maintain your weight, you'll need only 2,154 by the time you're 35; 2,110 at age 45: 2,068 at age 55: and so on.

The aging man's body replaces muscle with fat, which unfortunately burns fewer calories than muscle does. An adult man has less fat and about 10 to 20 percent more muscle than a woman of the same size and age does. Because muscle burns more calories than fat, a man's caloric needs are generally about 5 to 10 percent higher than a woman's.

Your metabolism:

Your body needs a minimum number of calories to maintain vital functions such as breathing and keeping your heart beating. This minimum number is called "Basal Metabolic Rate", or BMR. It's what we commonly refer to as "metabolism". You can compare your body to a car engine: some run efficiently, and others take a lot of fuel to run. A quick way to compute your BMR is to multiply your weight by 11. Your body needs approximately 11 calories per pound you weigh to meet its basic needs. Additional calories are needed for digestion and activity. For example, a 175-pound man needs about 1,925 calories. Genetics plays a part in determining your metabolic rate. That is why some men with the same height, weight and activity level are able to eat more calories than you do and not gain weight.

What is a Healthy Weight Range?

A healthy weight range is a range that relates statistically to good health. Health care professionals use three key measurements to determine whether you at a healthy weight:

Body Mass Index (BMI): A measure that correlates to how much fat is on your body.

Waist Size: A measure that indicates the location of your body fat.

Risk Factors for developing weight-related health problems: For example: your cholesterol level, blood pressure and family history.

To quickly estimate your healthy weight, you can use this method. First, figure the weight for your height using this formula:

106 pounds for 5 feet, plus 6 pounds per inch over 5 feet or minus 6 pounds per inch under 5 feet. You then calculate your range by

subtracting and adding 10 percent. You will be at the higher end of the range if you are a large-framed person or carry more muscle, and at the lower end of the range if you are small-framed with less muscle.

For example, if you are 6-feet-tall, your healthy weight range is 160-196 pounds.

Small-framed: 106 pounds plus 72 pounds minus 10 percent (about 18 pounds) = 160 pounds.

Large-framed: 106 pounds plus 72 pounds plus 10 percent (about 18 pounds) = 196 pounds.

You can also find your weight range using the *2010 Dietary Guidelines for Americans* weight table (see figure 1).

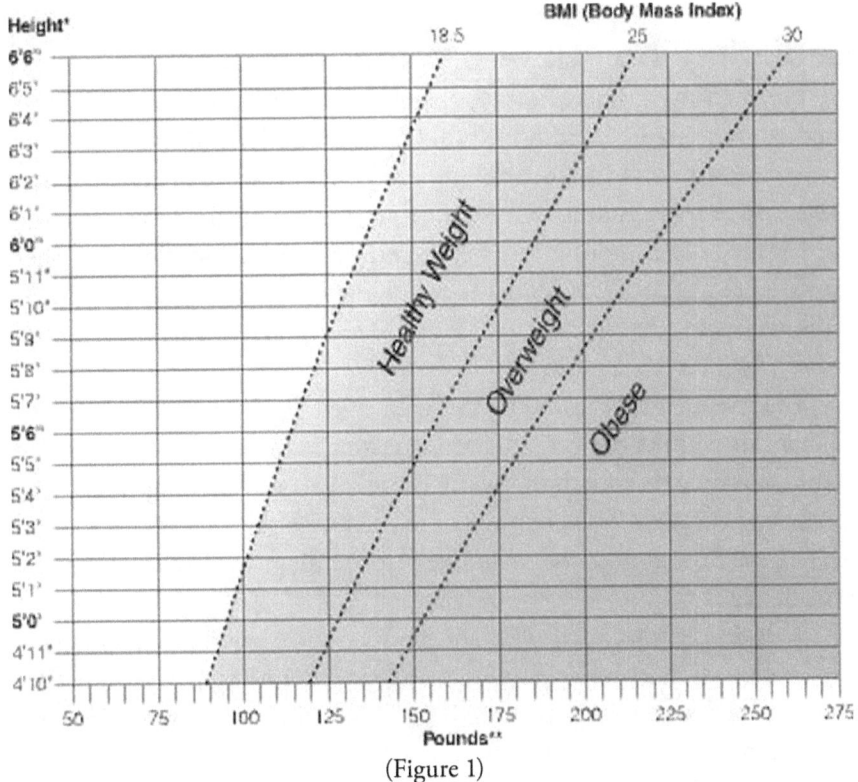

(Figure 1)

Source: Report of the Dietary Guidelines Advisory Committee on the Dietary Guidelines for Americans 2010, page 9.

Healthy Weight BMI from 18.5 up to 25 refers to healthy weight.

Overweight BMI from 25 up to 30 refers to overweight.

Obese BMI 30 or higher refers to obesity. Obese persons are also overweight.

BMI measures weight in relation to height. The BMI ranges shown above are for adults. They are not exact ranges of healthy and unhealthy weights. However, they show that health risk increases at higher levels of overweight and obesity.

Even within the healthy BMI range, weight gains can carry health risks for adults.

Directions: Find your weight on the bottom of the graph. Go straight up from that point until you come to the line that matches your height. Then look to find your weight group.

Reducing the risk of prostate cancer

For men over the age of 45, the threat of prostate cancer is a real concern. An article dated 8/30/2002 by Alan R. Kristal, DrPH, at the Cancer Prevention Center Program, Fred Hutchinson Cancer Research center in Seattle, stated that, " we found a strong link between the total amount of calories men took in and their risk of developing either localized or advanced prostate cancer". Kristal and colleagues published their study in the *Journal of Cancer Epidemiology, Biomarkers and Prevention* (Vol.II:719-725).

The researchers examined 1,197 men, aged 40-64, in the Seattle area to determine links between diet and prostate cancer. Men who ate the most calories had more than double the chance of being diagnosed with localized prostate cancer, compared to men who ate the fewest calories. They were also almost twice as likely to be diagnosed with advanced prostate cancer.

They found that men who ate the least fat-- less than 1/3 of their total calories- had half the risk of advanced prostate cancer of the others. They also found that men who took in more than 1200 mg of calcium daily, the amount in a quart of milk, had twice the risk of being diagnosed with advance prostate cancer compared to those who took in 500 mg daily.

Kristal suggested possible explanations for the study findings. Too many calories may raise blood sugar levels on insulin-like growth factors that promote rabid cell growth, raising chances of random error in DNA replication that could lead to cancer. And too much fat may raise levels of hormones that have similar effects on prostate cells. He added that calcium intake can help prevent thinning of the bones and lower the risk of coloncancer. But many studies have now shown a link between high calcium intake and the risk of prostate cancer. Some scientists believe that too much calcium may lower levels of a form of vitamin D that has anti-cancer properties.

Increasing your sexual activity has also shown to help in lowering your risk of developing prostate cancer (refer to chapter 7).

CHAPTER 4 - HEALTHY EATING GUIDES

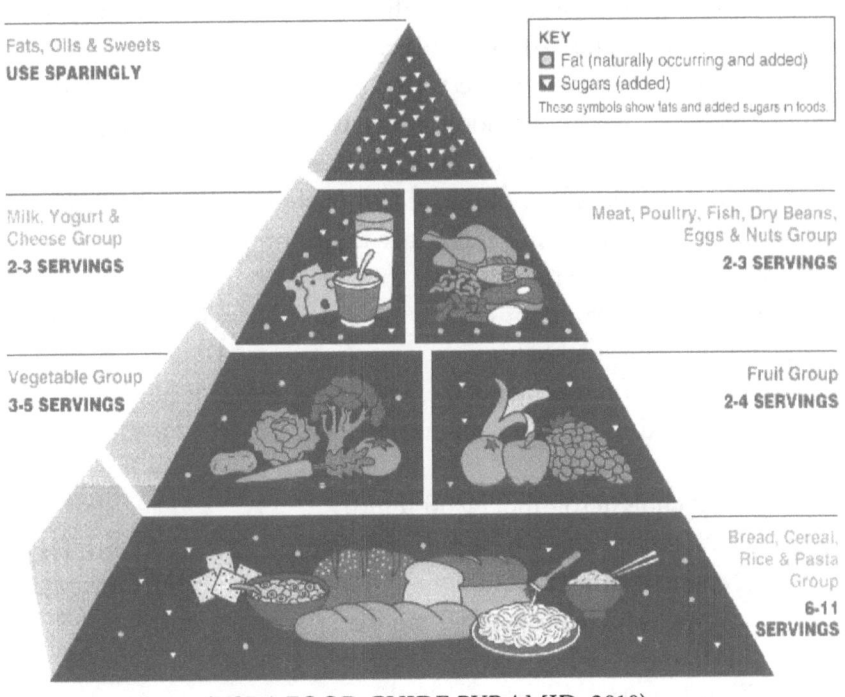

KEY
- Fat (naturally occurring and added)
- Sugars (added)

These symbols show fats and added sugars in foods.

Fats, Oils & Sweets
USE SPARINGLY

Milk, Yogurt &
Cheese Group
2-3 SERVINGS

Meat, Poultry, Fish, Dry Beans,
Eggs & Nuts Group
2-3 SERVINGS

Vegetable Group
3-5 SERVINGS

Fruit Group
2-4 SERVINGS

Bread, Cereal,
Rice & Pasta
Group
**6-11
SERVINGS**

(USDA FOOD GUIDE PYRAMID, 2010)

The Food Guide Pyramid provides a guideline for the various nutritional needs of children and adults. Most men fall into the mid-range with regard to the recommended intake of grains, fruits, vegetables, dairy, and protein. Some men feel that they need a larger amount of protein than is recommended based on strong activity levels. It's important to remember that exercise, not extra amounts of protein, builds muscle mass.

- Grain group: 9 servings per day
- Fruits: 2-3 servings per day
- Vegetables: 3-5 servings per day
- Meat: 2-3 servings per day
- Dairy: 2-3 servings per day
- Limit intake of fats and sugars

Remember that serving sizes are much smaller than we tend to think they are! Those numbers are not as high as you may think!

Calcium is important in not only helping with bone integrity but also with blood pressure. Some recent studies have also suggested a benefit with regard to weight loss. Although the majority of osteoporosis occurs in women, this issue also can affect men as well. So pay attention to your calcium intake—1000 milligrams per day.

Fruits, vegetables, and whole grains are full of antioxidants that can help decrease our risk of developing certain diseases, including cancer. Lycopene, found in tomatoes, may decrease the risk of developing prostate cancer. This is best obtained through cooked tomato products rather than raw. Fiber from these foods is also important in decreasing the risk of colon problems and heart disease.

Aim for 25-35 grams of dietary fiber per day, with at least 10 of these coming from soluble fiber.

Men should monitor their cholesterol levels as well as blood pressure levels with regard to the following guidelines:

- Total cholesterol under 200 mg/dL
- HDL greater than 40 mg/dL for men
  (Note that this is lower than the recommended HDL for women)
- Triglycerides less than 150 mg/dL
- LDL under 100 mg/dL
- Blood pressure less than 120/80

Talk to your doctor about a daily aspirin regimen. Much research has been done into the health benefits of a daily 81- milligram baby aspirin.

Men's weight should fall within healthy guidelines as well. A body mass index less than 25 is a good goal (18.5-24.9 is a healthy range). Most men tend to carry excess weight around the middle, which puts excess strain on the heart and is a higher risk factor for heart disease than weight that is carried around the hips. A good exercise regimen consists of at least 3 hours of aerobic exercise per week along with regular stretching and strength exercises. Be sure to vary your routine in order to avoid burnout and plateaus with regard to your weight loss goals.

If you supplement your intake with a multivitamin, look for one that is specially formulated for men. Most men's multivitamins will not contain iron. Don't take these on an empty stomach. Try this experiment to be sure that the one you are taking does actually break down in your body. Take half a cup warm water or vinegar and drop your vitamin in; wait 30 minutes (stirring at the 15 minute mark) and it should be fairly dissolved. If your supplement is hard as a rock at the end of 30 minutes, it's not breaking down in your system either! Also, be careful with overdoing the supplements as there is such a thing as too much. Supplements are not strictly regulated and we sometimes pay for more or less than what we think we are taking.

10 Easy Rules for Healthy Eating

Eat a minimum of 3 servings of vegetables and 2 servings of fruit each day.

Most men don't eat enough vegetables, especially the green leafy kind. Don't drink all your fruit as juices. Drinking fruit juice doesn't provide you with fiber and you will often drink more calories than you need. One serving of fruit equals about 4 ounces of juice.

Eat at Least 3 servings of whole grains each day.

20 to 35 grams of fiber per day are recommended. Whole wheat bread provides more fiber, vitamin E, vitamin B6, magnesium, zinc, copper, manganese and potassium than in white bread. The fiber difference between a slice of white bread and whole wheat is 2 grams.

Eat at least 4 servings of beans, lentils or peas each week.

Beans, lentils and peas are a good source of fiber and nutrients. These vegetables have enough protein to substitute for a serving of meat, fish or poultry.

Eat 3 meals and 2-3 small snacks a day.

We need to eat every 3 or 4 hours. Research has shown that people who snack often eat less than those who restrict their eating to the typical 3 meals a day. Your metabolism also works better when your body doesn't think it's starving.

Eat breakfast.

Missing breakfast is a big mistake. After an overnight fast, your body needs fuel to get going. This causes your metabolism to slow and reduces the number of calories you burn.

Limit soft drinks.

Soft drinks, especially the cola types have lots of caffeine, sugar and calories without any nutrients. Sugar-free versions don't add calories, but fat-free milk would be better because it is one of the best sources of calcium you can get.

Drink plenty of water.

The rule is about eight 8-ounce glasses a day. Humans are made up of 55 to 75 percent water. That's 10 to 12 gallons, depending upon body mass, age and sex. Men have more water because muscle holds greater amounts of water than fat. Also, the younger you are the greater the percentage of water. Studies have shown that when you think you are hungry, often you're actually thirsty, because dehydration is a major contributing factor to fatigue, which leads some people to seek food for energy. The average adult loses about 2 1/2 quarts of water a day: 4 to 6 cups in urine, 2 to 4 cups as perspiration, 1 1/2 cups through breathing and about 2/3 cup in feces. Roughly 3 to 4 1/2 cups of your daily water comes from food.

Limit caffeine to two servings or less a day.

Coffee is the main source of caffeine in the American diet, but tea, chocolate and cola drinks also contribute to a day's total amount. Caffeine speeds up your heart rate and can make you feel hyper and anxious. It can also contribute to dehydration due to its diuretic effect, which causes your body to lose water.

Limit salty foods.

The greatest source of salt in your diet comes from processed and prepared food. Eating lots of salt doesn't make you gain or lose weight, but it does cause water retention, which shows up temporarily as weight gains. You only need about 500 milligrams of sodium a day (about 1/4 teaspoon). Try keeping your salt intake to the advised levels of 2,400 milligrams or less a day. It takes only about 2 weeks to learn to enjoy the taste of unsalted food.

Limit the amount of saturated fat you eat.

Saturated fat contains the same number of calories as any other type of fat, but it raises your blood cholesterol level and increases your risk of heart disease. Animal products and topical oils (for example, palm and coconut) contain mainly saturated fat. As a general guideline, saturated fat is solid at room temperature. Examples include butter, stick margarine and the fat in meat and cheese.

Top 10 Best Foods For Men

Just as women need certain nutrients to protect themselves from osteoporosis, men need certain nutrients for prostate health. Men are also susceptible to suffering high levels of stress, more so than women, because they have a tendency to keep stress inside. And as in women, poor diet is a factor in heart disease for men, too. However, on average, men show signs of heart disease 10 to 20 years earlier than do women (although women are catching up due to high-stress related work environment).

The following is a list of the top 10 foods that will help men get healthier:

Tomatoes

Lycopene, the antioxidant is plentiful in tomatoes, is especially good in the prevention of prostate cancer. Even better doses of lycopene are found in cooked tomatoes, such as tomato sauce. More lycopene equals more protection. So the eating of spaghetti and pizza should be encouraged in the name of good health. Extra sauce please!

The President Liked Broccoli!

For men, broccoli is very helpful in the prevention of heart disease and cancer, the number one and number two killers of men over 35.

See The Seafood!

Seafood is high in protein and zinc. Zinc is important for immune function and (once again) prostate health. All men are at risk for prostate cancer over the age of 40. It may not sport a manly color, but that lovely pink salmon is filled to overflow with omega 3 fatty acids. Those fatty acids are effective in lowering the risk for prostate cancer. Salmon is also helpful for heart health, too.

Besides all that, salmon is on the women's list as well, so now you know what to order when you take that special someone out to dinner!

Garlic Protects Against More Than Vampires!

According to a study in Penn State's College of Health and Human Development, deodorized garlic capsules help bring down blood cholesterol levels of men. The men's cholesterol levels dropped 7 percent over 5 months, but remained unchanged in men downing placebos. But instead of swallowing pills, why not eat garlic in the food you love? Plus, garlic is also known for its aphrodisiac properties. What's not to like about garlic?

Time To Sow Your Oats!

Oatmeal is full of fiber, chock full of B vitamins (for stress), and contains lots of zinc for the prostate. If a hot bowl of oatmeal isn't your thing, you can do muffins.

The Rice Is Nice!

But don't chow down on just any style rice -- make it brown rice. Not only is it high in fiber, but it also has a good sampling of B vitamins, magnesium, potassium and zinc: all the stuff guys need.

Toss The Greens!

This is the stuff you loved to hate as a kid, but "gotta" eat as an adult. The experts say a whopping 35 percent of cancer deaths may be attributed to diet (it might even be more). Dark, leafy greens are nutrient-rich foods that are just packed with nutrition: beta-carotene, vitamin E, vitamin C, and important minerals such as calcium, magnesium and potassium. Get over the fear of greens and toss some down.

Be A Nut For Fruits!

Eaten raw, nuts are a great source of vitamin E, and adequate vitamin E helps maintain a healthy heart. Nuts are also filling and satisfying. Try a little raw almond butter on a piece of whole wheat bread with a half a banana sliced up on top. It's delicious! Bananas are a great portable fruit for everyone and they're a wonderful source of potassium, also important for a healthy heart.

Have A Thirst For Water!

It is estimated that as many as three out of four Americans are dehydrated! Water may not contain nutrition, but it is considered a nutrient because of the powerful effect it has on the body and bodily functions.

Ways to cut calories

Always Read The Nutrition Label On Packages

Buy the lower calorie items. Many product labels may sound healthy but may contain excess calories you don't need. Not all fat-free or reduced fat products are healthful from a caloric standpoint. Don't forget that!

Limit Your Alcohol

Alcohol may be fat free but has at least 7 calories per gram or about 70 calories per ounce (that's 2 tablespoons). The higher the proof, the more calories per ounce. Eighty proof alcohol has about 65 calories per ounce and 100 proof alcohol has about 85 calories per ounce. A light beer or a 5-ounce glass of wine contains about 100 calories. An average regular beer has about 150 calories.

Use A Smaller Plate

If you use a salad plate, about 8 inches in diameter, rather than a dinner plate, which is about 10-12 inches in diameter, your portions will be less and closer to the suggested portion size in the food pyramid.

Watch The Popcorn

The small popcorn at the movies contains about 150 calories. The large popcorn can contain over 1000 calories (that's without butter). A small soda (8 ounces) has about 95 calories, while a large soda (36 ounces or more) can have at least 400 calories.

Make a Plate In The Kitchen, Eat It In The Dining Room

If you fill up your plate and eat away from the food preparation, you will not be tempted to pick at extra food if the serving bowls are not right in front of you. You will be forced to go out of your way to get seconds.

Eat Off A Plate, Not Out Of The Box Or Bag

It's easier to limit your portions if you put a small amount onto your plate rather than eat out of the box or bag.

Cooking tips

If you are a man that likes or needs to cook, here are a few tips that will allow you to cook healthier. Remember the four B's: *barbecue, broil, bake or braise* and you will save a lot of calories over frying, stewing, or sautéing, because the fat has a chance to drip away from the meat thereby reducing the calories. Chicken and other poultry can be cooked with the skin on, removing it after cooking. Poultry doesn't absorb any additional fat, it just keeps the meat moist.

Sauté Onion And Garlic The Low Fat Way

Instead of cooking onions or garlic in oil, use a non-stick pan and 2 tablespoons of water in the place of oil. Use low heat and cover the pan to coax the natural juices out of the onion and garlic.

Make Your Own Vinaigrette Salad Dressing

You can reduce the standard vinaigrette salad dressing (one part vinegar to three parts oil) to one part oil, one part balsamic vinegar, and one part strong black tea or citrus juice such as orange or grapefruit. This will reduce the calories and give your salad dressing a nice flavor.

Roast The Vegetables

Since you need to eat more vegetables and steamed vegetables can be boring, Roast them in the oven. This will caramelize the natural sugars that they contain and add that extra flavor that steamed vegetables don't seem to have. Set your oven to 450°F. Slice the vegetables about 1/4 to 1/2 inch thick and arrange them in a single layer.

Coat them lightly with olive oil and roast them according to the times below:

-Carrots:	Roast for 15 to 20 minutes.
-Egg plant:	Roast for 10 to 15 minutes.
-Green Beans:	Roast for 12 minutes.
-Peppers:	Roast for 12 minutes.
-Onions:	Roast for 30 minutes.
-Sweet potatoes:	Roast for 15 minutes.
-Winter squash:	Roast for 8 to 10 minutes.
-Zucchini:	Roast for 5 to 8 minutes.

Use Fruit To Replace The Fat In Baked Foods

You can reduce the overall fat by replacing 1/4 of the fat using applesauce or apple butter or prune pie filling. This keeps the baked goods texture palatable.

Replace Bacon With Sun Dried Tomatoes

You can duplicate the smoky flavor that fatty pork adds to soups, salads and pizzas with chopped sun dried tomatoes. Don't use the oil packed ones. Soften up the dried tomatoes in a little hot water.

Substitute The Following Wherever You Can And Save Calories:

1 *medium sweet potato* for 1 *medium potato* and save 100 calories.
3 *ounces ground turkey* for 3 *ounces ground beef* and save 100 calories.
1 *cup fat free milk* for 1 *cup whole milk* and save 64 calories.
3 *ounces ground turkey* for 3 *ounces ground beef* and save 100 calories.
2 *egg whites* for 1 *whole egg* and save 46 calories.
3 1/2 *ounces tuna in water* for 3 1/2 *ounces tuna in oil* and save 80 calories.
1/2 *cup frozen yogurt* for 1 /2 *cup ice cream* and save 100 calories 1-cup 1% cottage cheese for 1-cup whole milk ricotta cheese and save 268 calories.

How to Shop and Dine

Shopping

Supermarkets are like giant booby traps for men, which is why if you send a man out to buy eggs, milk and bread you should not be surprised if he returns home with a case of wine, a pair of jeans and a canoe.

Going to the supermarket should be the time to stock up on healthy snacks in addition to the important foods needed. Remember the following tips when shopping to help you get only those foods and snacks you need to maintain a healthy lifestyle:

Always Make A Shopping List

This is always helpful so that you don't just wander through the store and buy things on impulse. The supermarket is laid out strategically to lure shoppers to pass through all the aisles in order to entice us buy the more expensive and non-essential items that we tend to buy impulsively such as cookies, candy and ice cream. That is why the more important stuff is located at the farthest points in the store like eggs, bread and vegetables.

Never Go Shopping On An Empty Stomach

Have a small snack before going to the store. Research has shown that people are less likely to purchase on impulse if they are not hungry when they shop. Being hungry makes a lot of those craved foods look too good to pass up.

Buy Single Serving Snacks

Buying individual servings instead of the big bag or box will help you eat smaller portions of snacks. This is better than sitting down and finishing a giant bag of chips or cookies. Food distributors want you to buy their "bargain" super-sized products. While this may make economic sense, you pay for it in overeating and excess calories.

Read The Label

The FDA (Food and Drug Administration) has mandated that all packaged foods must contain both ingredient and nutritional information on the package. Reading the label is important so that you know exactly what you are buying. The listing of the ingredients tells you how much proportionately each ingredient is in that particular package. The first listing has the most of that ingredient, while the last item listed has the least. For example, if the second ingredient listed is sugar, which means that the product has a higher proportion of sugar than the other ingredients. You must also be aware that the nutritional information listed is rated *per serving* and not based on the whole package.

Package design is sometimes used to mislead the public into thinking that the product being purchased is healthier than it truly is. For example, 2% fat reduced milk doesn't contain 2% fat as perceived. It means that there is 98% fat rather than 100% fat of whole milk. Only skim milk is fat free.

Carefully read the label of fat reduced products because a lot of times the reduced fat product may contain more sugar to make the product taste better to compensate for the texture lost in reducing the fat. This means that the reduced fat product has more calories than the regular version.

Dining out

Going to a restaurant should be a fun and relaxing experience. It's no fun when you have to worry about what you can or can't eat. Just understand that restaurants cater to the public's interest and not the betterment of people's health. Many restaurants, especially the cheaper ones, don't normally use low fat or low calorie cooking methods. The portions served in restaurants tend to be large and this contributes to overeating and taking in more calories than necessary. Waiting at the bar for our table, we usually have a drink and overindulge in eating only because we are paying a lot of money to dine out and want to get our money's worth.

Here are a few hints to eating out successfully:

Don't Be Afraid To Ask For A Doggy Bag

Restaurant meals are usually twice the amount you need to eat, so you don't have to finish everything on your plate. Eat half the meal and take the other half home for another meal. Or you can share the meal with your dining partner and overindulge in a salad bar.

Always Eat Your Meal Slowly

When you take your time to eat, your body will have the time to signal when your hunger is satisfied and you can stop eating. Don't loosen your belt! This is another way you can signal yourself that you have eaten enough.

Fast Food

Don't super-size your meals. For example: there is a major difference between a small French fry, which has approximately 210 calories and 10 grams of fat, and a super-sized one that can have as much as 540 calories and 26 grams of fat. A large 32-ounce soda has 310 calories, compared to 150 calories in a small one. Have a baked potato or rice instead of fries if you can. If you want to lose weight, have a kid's meal instead

Here Are A Few Rules To Follow When Dining Out:
1. Order broiled or baked instead of fried.
2. Have rice or a baked potato instead of fries.
3. Have extra vegetables instead of potato or bread.
4. Refrain from dishes that have a cheese or cream sauce.
5. Have your salad dressing on the side to control the amount.

Just remember that the easiest and cheapest ways that restaurants make their food taste better is by using a lot of fat. Ask questions about preparation and request substitutes. It's important that you don't use the excuse of eating out to over-indulge. Eat your meal within the context of what you ate for the entire day or what you will eat over several days.

PART 2 -
EXERCISE CAN BE FUN AND REWARDING

CHAPTER 5 - WHY EXERCISE IS SO IMPORTANT

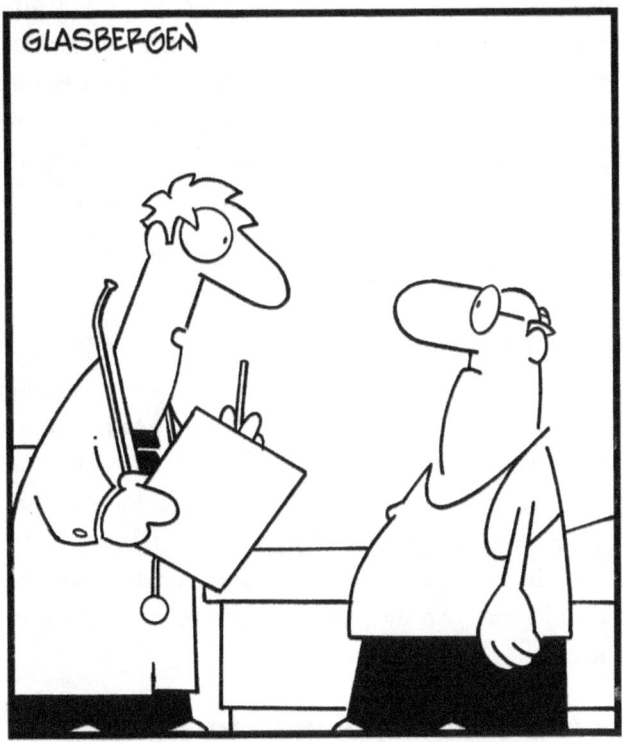

GLASBERGEN

"What fits your busy schedule better, exercising one hour a day or being dead 24 hours a day?"

Every doctor agrees that exercise is important to everyone. When you are fit you reduce the risk of having a heart attack or stroke, developing diabetes or some other crippling disease. The major benefits of exercise are as follows:

Exercise has psychological benefits:

Every time you exercise, you are doing something positive for yourself. So much of the weight-loss process involves giving up, limiting, and cutting out. But exercise is a positive addition, not a take away negative, and that's a powerful incentive for sticking with it. When you feel good about yourself, sticking to your weight-loss program is easy.

You eat less when you are busy or physically active:

The number one reason men eat is boredom, not because they are hungry. True hunger has little to do with why or how much you eat. This is why you mindlessly nibble on snacks while watching television. Some men believe that exercise makes them hungrier. This is just another excuse for not exercising. Fact: exercise helps slow the movement of food through your digestive tract. Your stomach takes longer to empty; therefore, you feel full longer. Fact: exercise uses the stored calories from the sugar and fat in your tissues so that the blood glucose levels stay even and you don't feel hungry.

Exercise burns calories:

The more calories you burn versus the amount of calories your body needs to maintain its current weight, the greater the weight loss. Another way that exercise helps burn calories is by increasing your metabolic rate--the rate which your body uses calories. Exercise helps you lose fat, not muscle, which determines how fast or slow your body burns calories. Muscle is active and needs more energy than fat, which is inert, to maintain itself. So the more muscle you have, the more calories your body needs.

Exercise protects against muscle loss:

When you diet, the weight that is lost is 75% fat and 25% muscle. This is not a good ratio. As muscle is lost so is your body's ability to burn and use calories efficiently. The less muscle and more fat is one of the reasons so many people on weight-loss diets restricting their calorie intake. who do not exercise reach a plateau and stop losing weight, even though they are still restricting their calorie intake

How much exercise is enough?

For weight loss, most experts agree that you need to expend a minimum of 200 to 300 calories a day for a minimum of 3 days a week. Research shows that for the best calorie burning, greater amounts of exercise at a lower intensity are better than high intensity for shorter periods. The following table shows some of the physical activities you can do to burn calories.

Calories Burned in 20 Minutes of Continuous Exercise

(BODY WEIGHT OF 185 LBS.)

ACTIVITY	CALORIES BURNED
BASKETBALL	136
GOLF (Carry Clubs)	184
TOUCH FOOTBALL	190
MOWING (Push Mower)	132
RAQUETBALL	212
JOGGING	212
DRIVING (Car)	64
SWIMMING	184
TENNIS	184
WALKING	84
* SEX (INCLUDING FOREPLAY)	172

Lose the Excuses and Start Exercising

Most men use the excuse that *"I don't have the time to exercise."* - This is just a cop out. You can always find the time to do the unimportant things you like, why not important ones?

Another excuse is *"I don't feel like it."* - You can get a buddy or several buddies and do your exercise together. Most men need the competition as motivation. Making a commitment to others helps and provides the support to keep going.

"I can't get to my gym to work out" – You don't need to belong to an expensive gym or workout place to get exercise. You can take the stairs, get off the train a few stops earlier and walk the rest of the way, park your car at the far end of the parking lot or walk up and down the station while waiting for the train.

"It hurts when I exercise" – Never exercise to the point of exhaustion. If you wake up stiff or in pain, slow down or cut back on the exercises

and slowly build up. If the activity doesn't feel good, don't do it! But you should get up every morning and do something.

Exercise doesn't have to be "all or none". You don't have to run a marathon or bench-press 500 pounds to get the necessary amount of exercise to get and stay in shape. Walking with your loved one every day can not only be good for your heart, but it can create a feeling of closeness and put your partner in a more receptive mood for other exercises.

How do you go from doing little to no exercise to developing a daily routine? Make it a habit. The easiest way to do this is to commit to exercise every day. Start with 20 minutes of daily walking. You can do two 10-minute walks if you like. Just commit to 20 minutes a day. After about two weeks, lengthen your walks to 40 minutes. In another two weeks, lengthen them to 60 minutes.

You don't have to do exercise all at once. It's the total daily amount that counts. It doesn't matter how you break it up as long as you get enough.

Eating tips for working out

If you can, eat 2 to 3 hours before working out because that's how long it takes for the meal to reach your muscles. Your body needs fuel, usually in the form of carbohydrates to get started. Try a bowl of cereal, a cup of low-fat yogurt or a banana. Always drink water to replace fluids, or you can drink a sports drink if you are exercising longer than an hour. Sports drinks are better than soda or fruit juice, which can upset your stomach during exercise and interfere with fluid absorption because they contain too much carbohydrate (about 12 to 15 percent by weight). Sports drinks contain 6 to 9 percent carbohydrates in the form of maltodextrins, sucrose and fructose. In addition, the small amounts of electrolytes, including sodium that sport drinks provide can replenish those lost through sweat.

CHAPTER 6 - EXERCISES TO LIVE BY

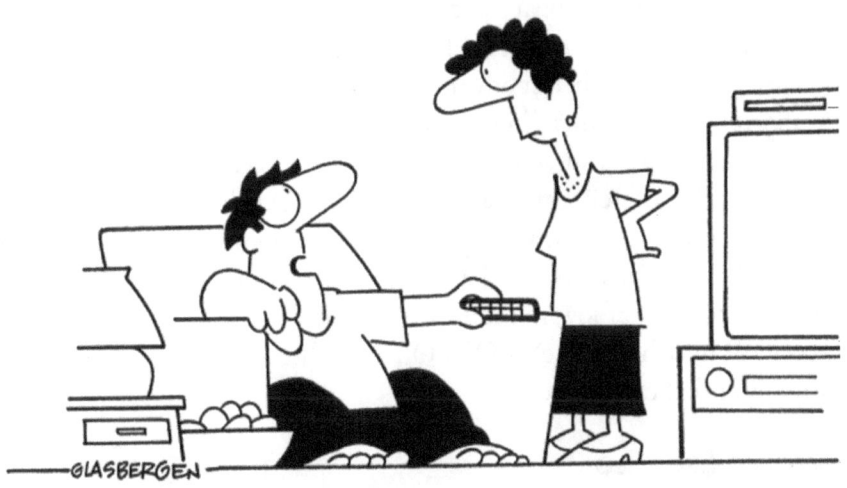

"Exercising builds muscle. Muscle makes you want to show off your body. To show off your body, you need a tan. Tanning turns your skin to leather. Cows are made of leather. Cows are fat. Therefore, exercising makes you fat!"

I love when I hear men say things such as "we won the soccer game" when they are really talking about how their kids' team won. Or the team they are rooting for on the TV wins, or when a man says he is going to walk the dog and stands in the backyard while the dog runs around. You're not engaged in a real activity. You are just being a spectator. Stop using active sounding phrases like "running to the store" when you are really driving your car. Or "mowing the lawn" and sitting on a mower.

Do something active like using the stairs instead of the elevator. Walk to talk to co-workers instead of e-mailing them. Have a catch with your kids instead of watching them play. Be a player not an on-looker. Active people lose weight more easily and tend to keep it off. As you start to exercise regularly you'll find it getting easier to add more strenuous types of exercises to your regimen. Again do not overdo it and hurt yourself. Moderation is the keystone to success. Focus first on increasing the length of time you exercise, then you can add a variety of activities such as weight training, jogging or stair climbing to a total of 60 minutes a day.

How Much Exercise And How Often?

Health benefits appear to be equal whether you do continuous aerobic exercise or intermittent. I prefer getting it all done at one time because you can take better advantage of a good warm-up. If you do opt for shorter walks or runs, they need to be at least 10-minute stretches of elevated heart rate, and you need to do at least 30 minutes combined.

An aerobic exercise program includes some dedicated aerobic time every day and strength training two to three times per week (no more frequently than every other day). On days you do strength training, 10 to 20 minutes of low to moderate aerobic activity (55 percent to 60 percent of max heart rate) is OK. On the other days, aim for 40 to 60 minutes of dedicated aerobics.

Aerobic Exercise

The strict definition of an aerobic exercise is *muscular movement that uses oxygen to burn both carbohydrates and fats to produce the energy needed to contract muscle cells.* During anaerobic exercise, muscle cells burn only carbohydrates to produce energy without using oxygen. For everyday purposes, aerobic exercise means repetitive muscular activity that causes the heart rate to accelerate and remain higher than usual over an extended period of time.

In general, you lose weight with prolonged aerobic exercise, while you build muscle strength with anaerobic exercise. The reality is that most recreational exercises, such as vigorous walking, running, swimming and cycling, are primarily aerobic. If you occasionally increase the pace and intensity, you will start to go anaerobic in some muscle groups. The reality is that you can't stay anaerobic for very long; it hurts too much from buildup of lactic acid, a normal byproduct of anaerobic metabolism. Anaerobic muscle activity will exhaust you in 60 seconds or less, often much less.

A commonly used indicator that you are staying aerobic is "the talk test" — simply the ability to talk while exercising. You may be breathing fast and hard, but if you can still carry on a conversation, you are still aerobic. If you are breathing so hard that you can't talk, you are more likely to be anaerobic. Failing the "talk test" lets you know that you may be going anaerobic.

Warming Up

Warm up for five to seven minutes for a 30- to 60-minute aerobic exercise routine. During these first few minutes your heart rate will increase quite quickly and then begin to level off. From here, the heart rate will tend to rise very gradually, assuming your workload remains constant or becomes slightly more strenuous. You have reached a steady state. The slow rise in heart rate from here is related to the normal increase in body temperature and release of "fight or flight" hormones from your adrenal glands (called catecholamines).

As you become more conditioned, you will experience a decrease in:
- Your resting heart rate
- How quickly your heart rate rises during the warm-up
- Your peak heart rate, even though you are working harder and longer than ever

The maximal heart rate declines with increasing aerobic fitness.

Walking:

Walking may be the perfect exercise: It's low-impact on joints and high-impact in results, burning as many calories on a per-mile basis as running (about 100 per mile for the average adult, although it obviously takes longer to cover that distance). It can be done anywhere at any time by just about anyone and requires no great athletic skills or special equipment other than a decent pair of shoes. And despite its reputation as being one of the more leisurely forms of exercise, it can offer a great total body workout. Here's how to make it even better:

Increase The Pace, Not The Stride:

Walking at a brisk 12- to 13- minute per mile pace (approximately 4.5 miles per hour) — achievable by most reasonably fit people — can substantially increase the aerobic benefits compared to walking at a pace of three miles per hour. Plus, you'll boost aerobic capacity faster than the slower 20-minute mile pace.

The Secret:

Take more steps per minute at your normal or a slightly shorter-than-normal stride, and don't increase your stride.

The Problem:

Many people take a bigger stride in an effort to cover more area in less time, but that only fatigues them more quickly.

The Advice:

Count off the steps you take in 60-second intervals and work to gradually increase the pace.

Line yourself up :

You may notice that Olympic and other elite race-walkers swing their hips more than recreational or beginning fitness walkers. That's because their feet move in a straight line, as opposed to walking with their legs at shoulder-width. This is called "railroading" because they walk as though they are on rails of a train track.

Walk Better:

Walk as if you drew a line on the ground, your left and right foot would be in that line. This causes you to swing your hips a bit more, which propels your body forward so you can walk at a faster rate.

Swing Those Arms Correctly:

The correct arm position is really the hands-on key to a better walking workout because it can actually propel the body forward, acting as something of a pendulum, and help you achieve a quicker and shorter stride. Arms should be bent at the elbow at an 85-degree angle and be pumping close to the body from the lower breast bone to the back of the hips.

The Mistake:

Some folks throw off their stride by either walking with straight arms and elbows locked, or allowing their arms to "chicken-wing" outward. And by moving your arms more quickly, you may also be able to boost your heart rate for a better workout.

Resistance Training:

Strength or resistance training, such as lifting weights or working out on exercise equipment, builds muscle. This type of exercise isn't just for body builders. Building muscle offers several benefits:

1. It gives your body definition and firmness.
2. It helps your body burn more calories.
3. It strengthens bones.

Working Out At Home

If you enjoy exercising by yourself at home, you're not alone. The home fitness industry is booming; Americans spend close to $1.7 billion on home equipment every year. Although working out at home can be both convenient and effective, the dropout rate for home exercisers is very high. So before purchasing a home gym, consider the following questions:

1. Will your roommates and/or family support your scheduled exercise time and not bother you?
2. Are you disciplined and motivated enough to exercise alone at regularly scheduled times?
3. Do you know how to exercise properly, and are you fully aware of the proper techniques for using home fitness equipment?

Evaluating Exercise Equipment

After you've made the decision to work out at home, the most important consideration is to be realistic about buying your equipment. Too many people purchase expensive exercise bikes or treadmills, work out on them for a few weeks and then use them for hanging clothes. Before making any substantial investment in a piece of equipment — whether it's a bike, treadmill, stair climber or skiing machine — try out a similar device at a health club or gym for a month or two (using a guest pass or a temporary membership) to make sure it can hold your interest for 30 minutes or more. Some manufacturers also offer a free trial period.

The other important factors to consider are how well the machine functions and how it holds up over time. Avoid cheaper models by lesser-known companies — a well-made, leading brand will be worth the extra cost because it should last for many years.

Exercise Bikes

The seat should be padded and adjustable. The bike should be able to challenge but not exhaust you, and it should ride smoothly and quietly. You should be able to vary the level of exercise easily. Recumbent bikes are good for people with lower back problems.

Treadmills

A quality unit should have 1.5 horsepower or more, and the deck size (minimum 25 inches wide and 65 inches long) should accommodate your walking and running stride. You should be able to vary the speed and incline easily, and the treadmill should run fairly quietly.

Cross Country Ski Machines

The machine should have a solid construction, independent arm-lever action and a smooth sliding action. You should be able to easily adjust the resistance and the angle of incline without dismounting. The machines with bi-directional resistance are easier to use than the flywheel and pulley-type units.

Stair Climbers

The unit should be solid and stable and have a smooth stepping action. You will get a better workout from stair climbers with independent foot action.

Other Tips:

- Invest in a floor mat (available in sporting goods stores) for stretching exercises.
- If you plan to do strength training with free weights, adjustable weight dumbbells with metal plates are the preferred choice because they're easier to manage than barbells. If you prefer weight machines, your best bet is still a health club, which offers a variety that can't easily be matched in a home gym.
- -If you have the room, try to set up an area exclusively for exercise. This added convenience will boost your motivation to work out.
- If you purchase an aerobic device for home use, don't rely exclusively on it. To make workouts less boring, mix some stationary aerobic exercise with some walking, running or cycling (You can alternate

days — or do 20 to 25 minutes of one activity, then switch to another).

And don't forget the most important exercise you can do is sex! Besides being the most enjoyable physical activity a man can do, the long-term health benefit is not to be made light of. The next chapter points out all the health benefits that a good sex life brings to you.

In order to have the type of relationship with your significant other that will allow you to have sex that many times a week, your relationship must be a close one. In order for your relationship to be that close, you must learn to communicate and understand each other better.

Parts 3 and 4 of this book will focus on how you can improve your relationship and reduce your stress.

This creates a balanced lifestyle combining healthy eating, exercising, having more sex and reducing stress.

CHAPTER 7 - IMPORTANCE OF SEXUAL ACTIVITY FOR HEALTH REASONS

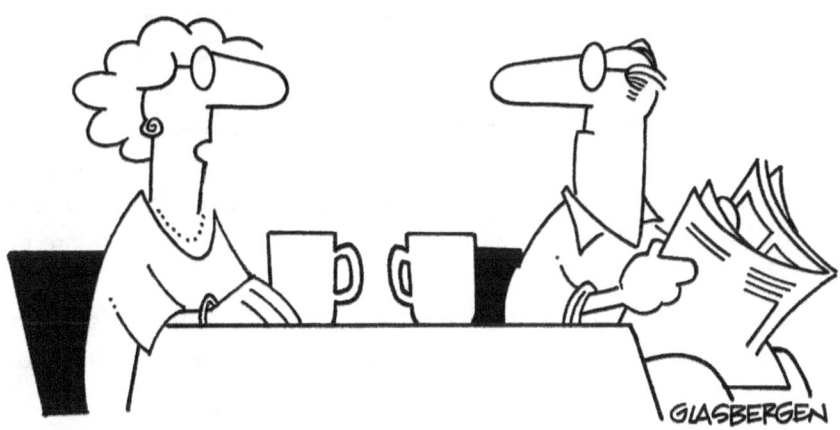

**"Same-sex marriage is nothing new.
We've been having the same sex for 25 years."**

Besides being the most enjoyable activity for both men and women, sex has many benefits for men in terms of long range health. A great deal of research points to the benefits of social interaction and social support in helping heart health. While there are many different types of relationships that are supporting, the relationship with a partner willing to be intimate multiple times a week has more longer lasting effects than "one night stands".

Sex is good for your health. Most people enjoy sex for its own sake, but a study suggests that men who have sex at least three times a week cut their risk of a heart attack in half.

Researchers started out studying the benefits of vigorous exercise, looking at an activity lasting 20 minutes or longer and making the exerciser sweaty or out of breath. Most of the men they questioned thought that sex fit this description just as well as soccer.

This surprised the scientists, but they decided to study the issue.

About 2,400 men in the town of Caerphilly in South Wales were questioned about their habits, including how often they had sex—once, twice or three times a week or more. Then they were followed up for ten years. Those who reported the most frequent sexual activity were only half as likely to suffer a stroke or heart attack during that time.

The doctors conducting the study concluded that intercourse is good exercise. Other research has shown that even walking briskly for 20 minutes at least three times a week can help ward off such cardiovascular crises, so that explanation may be adequate. But there may even be something else at work.

A great deal of research points to the benefits of social interaction and social support in helping heart health. While many different types of relationships may be supportive, the relationship with a partner willing to engage in sex three times a week or more often is likely to be very close indeed.

Promiscuity isn't likely to have such health benefits. Japanese scientists recently announced that people engaging in adulterous relations were more susceptible to fatal strokes.

A loving and sexually fulfilling relationship is not always easy to achieve. People are so over-committed these days that taking time out of a busy schedule to enjoy sexuality may seem like a challenge. This is especially true for people on medications that may interfere with libido or the ability to climax.

So Just What Health Benefits Does Sex Bring?

Reduced risk of heart disease:

For men! Having sex 3 to 4 times a week will cut your risk of heart attack or stroke in half! Women also benefit in this category though the results are not as clear in percentage.

Overall fitness:

During sex, the average person maintains his/her heart rate above 70% of the maximum, making sex a wonderful workout.

Reduced depression:

Sperm contains prostaglandin (a male sex hormone), that when absorbed in the female reproductive tract helps to regulate female hormones in maintaining a balance and decreasing mood swings and depression.

Pain relief:

Endorphins released immediately upon orgasm are natural pain relievers that remain active in the body for several hours after climaxing. Intercourse also produces more estrogen in the female body, which helps to reduce the discomfort of monthly PMS.

Improved immunity:

People who have sex once or twice a week have been shown to have higher rates of immunoglobulin A, a known immune booster.

Better bladder control:

The muscles used during sex are the same used in doing the infamous "kegel exercises". Yes, this applies to men too!

Improved sense of smell:

Prolactin (a hormone produced after sex) stimulates the olfactory nerve, the center for smell, thus increasing smell perception.

Nicer teeth:

Seminal fluid contains zinc, calcium and minerals that retard tooth decay! So for the girls', going down isn't just fun for her and great for him, it's an awesome way to put a great smile on both your faces!

If size counts:

A great side effect of weight loss is that losing 25 to 30 pounds can decrease the amount of fat situated at the base of your penis. This fat loss, believe it or not, can actually add up to an inch to the length of your penis.

A happier prostate:

To produce seminal fluid, the prostate and the seminal vesicles take minerals, zinc, and calcium and concentrate them up to 600 times.

However, any carcinogens in the blood would also be concentrated to this amount. Urologists support ejaculation as a measure of prostate cancer prevention by removing the concentrated carcinogens rather than allowing them to cluster and cause damage.

Long Term Health Benefits

The long-term health benefits of an intimate and nurturing relationship should not be underestimated. Many relationships suffer from a tendency to accept denial of both physical and emotional needs being met and maintained throughout the relationship. Men begin to take their partner for granted and they no longer pay attention to the details of the relationship that made it work when they were in pursuit of their mate. Some men become complacent about having a limited amount of sex.

This occurs primarily because their partner is not receiving the emotional support to foster an interest in intimacy and sexual fulfillment. This tends to lead to certain men having their sexual needs met in socially unacceptable solutions (infidelity, one-night stands, prostitutes and divorce).

This is the main contributing factor for a belief in the " mid-life crisis" phenomenon in men (refer to chapter 8).

CHAPTER 8 - THE MID LIFE CRISIS

The Mid Life Crisis Is Really Male Menopause

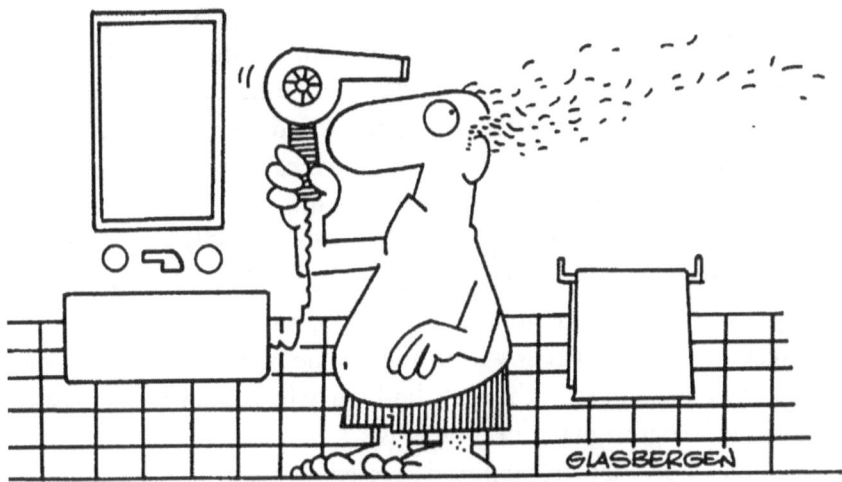

**Glen can tell you the exact moment
that his midlife crisis began.**

What is Male Menopause?

"Male menopause is a lot more fun than female menopause," a female comedian once said. "With female menopause you gain weight and get hot flashes. With male menopause you get to date young girls and drive motorcycles."

While not entirely true in the latter aspect, her statement only serves to highlight the haze surrounding the condition. Male menopause (also called *viropause* or *andropause*) begins with hormonal, physiological, and chemical changes that occur in all men generally between the ages of forty and fifty-five, though it can occur as early as thirty-five or as late as sixty-five.

Unlike women (who cannot get pregnant after menopause), men can continue to father children, but the production of the male sex hormone (testosterone) diminishes gradually after age 40. Testosterone is the hormone that stimulates sexual development in the male infant, and bone and muscle growth in adult males. It is also responsible for sexual drive. It has been found that even in healthy men, by the age of 55 the amount of testosterone secreted into the bloodstream is significantly lower than it is just 10 years earlier. In fact, by age 80 most male hormone levels decrease to pre-puberty levels.

These changes affect all aspects of a man's life. Male menopause is, thus, a physical condition with psychological, interpersonal, social and spiritual dimensions. The purpose of male menopause is to signal the end of the first part of a man's life and prepare him for the second half. Male menopause is not the beginning of the end, as many fear, but the end of the beginning. It is the passage to the most passionate, powerful, productive, and purposeful time of a man's life.

While there is much dispute both over the validity of potential causes and the recommended treatment of the condition known as male menopause, there is no doubt that changes occur within the male body as it ages, just as they occur within the female body. It is also possible that hormonal changes in the male body may be primarily responsible for the mythological male "mid-life crisis".

Fatigue, depression, irritability, decreased libido, erectile dysfunction, pain, stiffness and hair loss have all been ascribed as symptoms of male menopause. Many physicians point to decreased testosterone production as men age as the factor responsible for the onset of this condition, similar to the drop in estrogen levels experienced by women during menopause. For women, however, the changes tend to be more abrupt. Men tend to experience a slower decline in testosterone levels.

How can a man tell if he's headed for the dreaded *"andropause"*?

Certain classical symptoms can alert a person to the fact that subtle changes are taking place in his body, and he should change his lifestyle accordingly.

Sexual:
- Reduced interest in sex
- Increased anxiety and fear about losing sexual potency
- Increased fantasies about having sex with a new and younger partner
- More relationship problems and fights over sex, love, and intimacy
- Loss of erection during sexual activity

Physical:
- Taking longer to recover from injuries and illness
- Less endurance for physical activity
- Feeling fat, gaining weight
- Difficulty reading small print
- Loss or thinning of hair
- Sleep disturbances

Psychological:
- Irritability
- Indecisiveness
- Anxiety and fear
- Depression
- Loss of self-confidence and joy
- Loss of purpose and direction in life
- Feeling lonely, unattractive, and unloved
- Forgetfulness and difficulty concentrating

Causes.
Although all the causes of male menopause have not been fully researched, some factors that are known to contribute to this condition are hypothalamic sluggishness, hormone deficiencies, excessive alcohol consumption, obesity, smoking, hypertension, prescription and non-prescription medications, poor diet, lack of exercise, poor circulation, psychological problems and notably mid-life depression. A general decline in potency at mid-life can be expected in a significant proportion of the male population. A relative increase in circulating levels of estrogen (which competes with testosterone for cellular receptor sites) can tilt the testosterone- estrogen balance unfavorably and can reduce the availability of testosterone to target cells.

Hormones, Male PMS and Health Problems
Hormonal changes greatly affect men going through male menopause. Lowered levels of hormones at mid-life are central to the changes associated with male menopause. Recent research indicates that lowered levels of dopamine, oxytocin, vasopressin, growth hormone, melatonin, DHEA, pregnenolone, thyroid hormone, and testosterone

may decrease sex drive, increase depression and weight gain, and contribute to a general decrease in well being and health.

Although these hormones tend to decrease with age, each man is unique, and individual levels vary widely. Men have physical and emotional reactions to hormonal fluctuations throughout the month, similar to PMS in a woman.

In a recent study, when men were given the same checklists of symptoms from a typical PMS questionnaire (omitting the female specific symptoms such as breast tenderness), men reported having as many premenstrual type symptoms as women do (reduced energy, irritability, and other negative moods, back pain, sleeplessness, headaches, confusion, etc).

Treatment:

Hormone replacement therapy can be prescribed, especially in severe cases of testosterone deficiency. It is, however, estimated that testosterone deficiency accounts for less than ten per cent of all cases of erectile dysfunction. Men should be aware that there is some concern that increased levels of testosterone may increase the risk of prostate cancer and heart disease. Your physician can advise you about the pros and cons of hormone replacement therapy.

Sex and Aging

It is a common belief that as you get older, you lose your sex drive and sexual intimacy is no longer an option. This is a myth, and an extremely erroneous one at that. A person's sex drive may experience some changes as a result of many factors, but it does not necessarily disappear. The factors that affect sex-drive are psychological and physiological in nature. As a rule of thumb, if you have a healthy sex drive when you're young, you will continue to have a healthy drive well into your senior years; however, if you're not very active in your twenties, you can't expect a dramatic change without a lot of work and motivation.

Sexual Changes with Age

The primary physiological changes that occur in both men and women are due to the change in hormone levels; testosterone levels in men and estrogen levels in women. The gradual decrease in these hormones causes a variety of changes in the physical ability to perform sexually; however, these changes can be overcome with time, patience and communication.

Physiological Changes in Men

For men, these physical changes occur over a period of time. As a man ages, there is a decrease in the amount of circulating testosterone; this stabilizes by about 60 years of age. As a result of this decrease in testosterone levels, it will take a man much longer to achieve a full erectile state. At a young age, a man is able to obtain an erection with visual and mental stimulation; however, as a man ages, he will need more direct manual stimulation in order to achieve the same affect.

There is also a decrease in the length of time a man is able to maintain an erection prior to ejaculation. This is due to a variety of other physical factors that affect blood flow: hypertension, diabetes, and cardiac arrhythmia, to name a few. There is also a decrease in the force of ejaculation due to a reduction in the sperm count. The refractory phase of sexual intercourse is also lengthened. It will take a man much longer to have the ability to have another orgasm, usually 12 to 24 hours. This time period increases as a man continues to age.

Another very important fact to remember is the following: If a man discontinues sexual activity in his fifties to sixties, he will have a much greater chance of having impotency problems. If he continues sexual activity, the chances of impotency are far less. Just remember "use it or lose it".

PART 3 –
HEALTHY LIVING THROUGH
A BETTER RELATIONSHIP

CHAPTER 9 - HOW TO BUILD A BETTER RELATIONSHIP

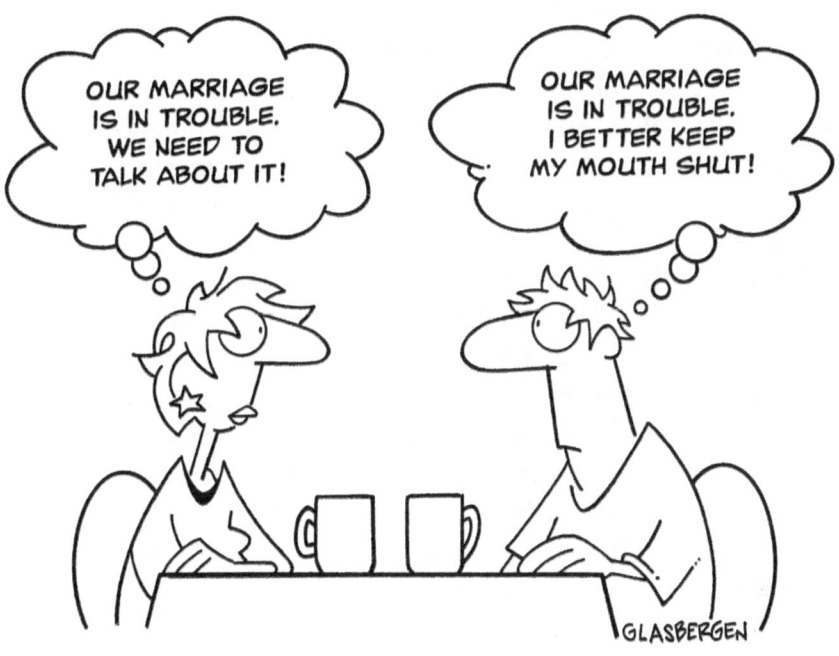

"Women can use sex to get what they want,
Men can't, because sex is what they want!"

In order to have a more intimate relationship with your significant other, you must learn to communicate with each other. Remember when you were first dating? How good the sex was and how often! Then one day the relationship changed. Both partners focused on work, children, paying bills and less time on tending to each other's needs. One of the things that changed is the amount of stress we allow ourselves to have. Stress and fatigue are the chief culprits in squashing sexual desire. Stress releases chemicals into the brain that are known to dampen sexual desire, while tiredness can lead to sex that is unsatisfying and boring.

Ira Epstein

The Differences Between Men and Women:

"Women have their faults. Men have only two.
Everything they say and everything they do."

For centuries, the differences between men and women were socially defined and distorted through a lens of sexism in which men assumed superiority over women and maintained it through domination. As the goal of equality between men and women now grows closer we are also losing our awareness of important differences. In some circles of society, politically correct thinking is obliterating important discussion as well as our awareness of the similarities and differences between men and women. The vision of equality between the sexes has narrowed the possibilities for discovery of what truly exists within a man and within a woman. The world is less interesting when everything is the same.

It is my position that men and women are equal but different. When I say "equal", I mean that men and women have a right to equal opportunity and protection under the law. The fact that people in this country are assured these rights does not negate the observation that men and women are at least as different psychologically as they are physically.

None of us would argue the fact that men and women are physically different. The physical differences are rather obvious and most of these can be seen and easily measured. Weight, shape, size and anatomy are not political opinions but rather tangible and easily measured. The physical differences between men and women provide functional advantages and have survival value. Men usually have greater upper body strength, build muscle easily, have thicker skin, bruise less easily and have a lower threshold of awareness of injuries to their extremities. Men are essentially built for physical confrontation and the use of force. Their joints are well suited for throwing objects. A man's skull is almost always thicker and stronger than a women's is. The stereotype that men are more "thick-headed" than women is not far-fetched. A man's "thick headedness" and other anatomical differences have been associated with a uniquely male attraction to high speed activities and reckless behavior that usually involve collisions with other males or automobiles. Men, not women, invented the game of "chicken". Men, and a number of other male species of animal, seem to charge and crash into each other a great deal in their spare time.

Women, on the other hand, have four times as many brain cells (neurons) connecting the right and left side of their brain. This latter finding provides physical evidence that supports the observation that men rely easily and more heavily on their left brain to solve one problem one step at a time. Women have more efficient access to both sides of their brain and therefore greater use of their right brain. Women can focus on more than one problem at one time and frequently prefer to solve problems through multiple activities at a time. Nearly every parent has observed how young girls find the conversations of young boys "boring". Young boys express confusion and would rather play sports than participate actively in a conversation among 5 girls who are discussing as many as three subjects at once!

The psychological differences between men and women are less obvious. They can be difficult to describe. Yet these differences can profoundly influence how we form and maintain relationships that can range from work and friendships to marriage and parenting.

Recognizing, understanding, discussing as well as acting skillfully in light of the differences between men and women can be difficult. Our failure to recognize and appreciate these differences can become a life-long source of disappointment, frustration and tension, and will eventually lead to our downfall in a relationship. Not only can these differences destroy a promising relationship, but also most people will grudgingly accept or learn to live with the consequences. Eventually they find some compromise or way to cope. Few people ever work past these difficulties. People tend to accept what they don't understand when they feel powerless to change it.

Relationships between men and women are not impossible or necessarily difficult. Problems simply arise when we expect or assume the opposite sex should think, feel or act the way we do. It's not that men and women live in completely different realities. Rather, our lack of knowledge and mutual experience gives rise to our difficulties.

Despite great strides in this country toward equality, modern society hasn't made relationships between men and women any easier. Today's society has taught us and has imposed on us the expectation that men and women should live together continuously, in communion and in harmony. These expectations are not only unrealistic but ultimately they leave people feeling unloved, inadequate, cynical, apathetic or ashamed.

The challenge facing men and women is to become aware of their identities, to accept their differences, and to live their lives fully and as skillfully as possible. To do this we must first understand in what ways we are different. We must avoid trying to change others to suit our needs. The following illustrates some important differences between men and women. These differences are not absolute. They describe how men and women are in most situations most of the time.

Problems

"When faced with flat-packed furniture, men never read the manual, yet they spend hours reading manuals for cars or bikes they will never own!"

Men and women approach problems with similar goals but with different considerations. While men and women can solve problems equally well, their approach and their process are often quite different. For most women, sharing and discussing a problem presents an opportunity to explore, deepen or strengthen the relationship with the person they are talking with. Women are usually more concerned about how problems are solved than merely solving the problem itself. For women, solving a problem can profoundly impact whether they feel closer and less alone or whether they feel distant and less connected. The process of solving a problem can strengthen or weaken a relationship. Most men are less concerned and do not feel the same as women when solving a problem.

Men approach problems in a very different manner than women. For most men, solving a problem presents an opportunity to demonstrate their competence, their strength of resolve, and their commitment to a relationship. How the problem is solved is not nearly as important as solving it effectively and in the best possible manner. Men have a tendency to dominate and to assume authority in a problem solving process. They set aside their feelings, provided the dominance hierarchy was agreed upon in advance and respected. They are often distracted and do not pay attention to the quality of the relationship while solving problems. Try talking to a man while he is working on a project and you will see what I mean.

Some of the more important differences can be illustrated by observing groups of young teenage boys and groups of young teenage girls when they attempt to find their way out of a maze. A group of boys generally establish a hierarchy or chain of command with a leader who emerges on his own or through demonstrations of ability and power. Boys explore the maze using scouts while remaining in distant proximity to each other. Groups of girls tend to explore the maze together as a group without establishing a clear or dominant leader. Relationships tend to be co-equal. Girls tend to elicit discussion and employ "collective intelligence" to the task of discovering a way out. Girls tend to work their way through the maze as a group. Boys tend to search and explore using structured links and a chain of command.

Thinking

"A successful man is one who makes more money than his wife can spend. A successful woman is one who can find such a man."

While men and women can reach similar conclusions and make similar decisions, the process they use can be quite different, and in some cases can lead to entirely different outcomes. In general, men and women consider and process information differently.

Women tend to be intuitive global thinkers. They consider multiple sources of information within a process that can be described as simultaneous, global in perspective, and will view elements in the task in terms of their interconnectedness. Women come to understand and consider problems all at once. They take a broad or "collective" perspective, and they view elements in a task as interconnected and interdependent. Women are prone to become overwhelmed with complexities that "exist", or may exist, and may have difficulty separating their personal experience from problems.

Men tend to focus on one problem at a time or a limited number of problems at a time. They have an enhanced ability to separate themselves from problems and minimize the complexity that may exist. Men come to understand and consider problems one piece at a time. They take a linear or sequential perspective, and view elements in a task as less interconnected and more independent. Men are prone to minimize, and fail to appreciate subtleties that can be crucial to successful solutions. A male may work through a problem repeatedly, talking about the same thing over and over rather than trying to address the problem all at once.

While there are differences in the ways that men and women think, it must be emphasized that they can and do solve problems in a similar manner. There are no absolutes, only tendencies.

Memory

> *"A woman worries about the future until she gets a husband while a man never worries about the future until he gets a wife."*

Women have an enhanced ability to recall memories that have strong emotional components. They can also recall events or experiences that have similar emotions in common. Women are very adept at recalling information, events or experiences in which there is a common emotional theme. Men tend to recall events using strategies that rely on reconstructing the experience in terms of elements, tasks or activities that took place. Profound experiences that are associated with competition or physical activities are more easily recalled. There appears to be a structural and chemical basis for observed memory differences. For instance, the hypocampus, the area in the brain primarily responsible for memory, reacts differently to testosterone in men and it reacts differently to changing levels of estrogen and progesterone in women. Women tend to remember or be reminded of different "emotional memories" and content to some extent as part of their menstrual cycle.

Sensitivity

> *"A woman marries a man expecting he will change, but he doesn't. A man marries a woman expecting that she won't change and she does".*

There is evidence to suggest that a great deal of the sensitivity that exists within men and women has a physiological basis. It has been observed that is many cases, women have an enhanced physical alarm response to danger or threat. Their autonomic and sympathetic systems have a lower threshold of arousal and greater reactivity than men. In both men and women, higher levels of testosterone directly affect the aggressive response and behavior centers of the brain. Increasing estrogen and progesterone in men has a "feminizing" effect. Sexually aggressive males become less focused on sexual aggressive behavior and content when they are given female hormones. On the other hand, changing estrogen and progesterone levels in women during menstrual cycles can produce a "flood" of memories as well as strong emotions. Increasing or high levels of testosterone can produce an emotional insensitivity, empathic block and increased indifference to the distress others.

At the heart of sensitivity is our capacity to form, appreciate and maintain relationships that are rewarding. Even here there are important differences. For men, what demonstrates a solid relationship is quite different from that of most women. Men feel closer and validated through shared activities. Such activities include sports, competition, outdoor activities or sexual activities that are decidedly active and physical. While both men and women can appreciate and engage in these activities, they often have preferential differences. Women, on the other hand, feel closer and validated through communication, dialogue and intimate sharing of experience, emotional content and personal perspectives. Many men tend to find such sharing and involvement uncomfortable, if not overwhelming.

Relationships Between Men and Women

"To women love is an occupation. To men it is a preoccupation."

The task that faces men and women is to learn to accept their differences, avoid taking their differences as personal attempts to frustrate each other, and to compromise whenever possible. The idea that one gender can think and feel like the other if they truly loved each is rather absurd. Sure, a man or woman could act in consideration of the other's needs, but this would not necessarily be rewarding and honest. Holding the benefit of another above our own is rewarding. But from time to time, and more often for most of us, it is important to be ourselves and to be accepted, and not to be the source of distress and disappointment in the lives of people we love.

Communication Between Men and Women

*"When women are depressed they either eat or go
shopping. Men invade another country."*

Remember where we came from. In certain ways men are still hunters from a prehistoric age. Just as they will not ask for directions when driving their car, or using the remote control for the television set like a spear, while hunting for a program to watch.

Men get frustrated and angry when they do not have control over what is happening to them. They need to be in control of their emotions, and when they are not, they feel guilty. In comparison, women get angry or stressed about problems they are having in their most intimate relationships.

Men and women also communicate differently. Women will articulate their thought process as they are going through it before making a final decision, while men will internalize the same process and only verbalize the end result. That is why men accuse women of changing their minds all the time, while women accuse men of not considering an issue or not caring

According to relationship counselor John Gray, difficulties in relationships between a man and a woman lie in the lack of understanding and acceptance of the differences between the two sexes. Gray's famous book *Men Are From Mars, Women Are From Venus* turned out to be a phenomenal best seller. Since its initial print in 1992, over 11 million copies were sold in the U.S. alone. In addition, it was translated into 40 different languages and has readers all over the world. To many, Gray has achieved guru status in the fields of communication and relationships. To some others, however, Gray's Mars-Venus model stereotypes both men and women. In particular, he has been accused of having pushed women's role in marriage back 30 years. To the author, the book *Men Are From Mars, Women Are From Venus* portrays men or women in neither a good nor a bad light, but in true light. It may make men or women sound like a good or bad deal to their partners, but according to the book it is the only deal we get. Therefore, acknowledgment and acceptance are key.

Now, let's take a look at the differences between men (Martians) and women (Venusians) as they are depicted in Dr. Gray's book.

- Men like to help women by fixing problems.
- Women like to help men by improving men.
- Men do not like women's attempt to improve them. They feel humiliated.
- Fixing problems for them is not what women want the most from men.
- When men are down, they want women's loving acceptance, not their criticism and unsolicited advice.
- Men want to be trusted and admired.
- When women are down, they like to talk about their problems. They want men to be sympathetic listeners, not necessarily offer solutions to their problems.
- Men are goal-oriented problems solvers.
- Women have a need to talk about their feelings. They need to be heard and understood. Instead of being busy figuring out how to solve their problems. Men should show their acknowledgment vocally or through nodding and brief eye contact.
- Men talk to exchange information.
- Women talk to express feelings.
- Men need to be alone sometimes. Every now and then, especially when under stress, they need to retreat to their "cave" and do not want to be disturbed. Insisting on helping them before they are ready to emerge from the cave can feel like harassment.
- Women, under stress and in other times, like to seek out contact and make human connections.
- Naturally and cyclically, women's moods go through highs and lows.
- Men are often disconcerted by women's emotions.
- Women tend to use dramatic expressions such as "you ALWAYS forget" or "you NEVER listen to me". Men should not take those literally but sympathize with the sentiments they convey.
- Men and women, even when they speak the same words, may speak different languages.

Differences Between Men and Women in Conversation

"When men want something, they ask for it. When women want something they make a point distantly related to the subject and wait for a response."

In my opinion, one of the most beneficial areas of research has been the studies of conversations between males and females. In brief, this research indicates that the young boy-girl interaction styles described in the problem section continue for a lifetime in our male-female conversational styles. Men and women operate in two very different social worlds. Men are in an ongoing contest, competing with everyone by displaying their competence and skill. Why don't men ask for directions when lost? Because it puts them in a "you-know-more-than-I-do" position. Women are cautious but persistently seek intimacy; they want emotional support, cooperation, and praise. Given these different orientations, it is no wonder that the sexes have trouble communicating!

If both sexes understand where the other is "coming from," however, the conflicts can be reduced. Examples: a man can gain an understanding of how his wife can love talking on and on to her female friends about a problem and never receive any advice or criticism. The women are interacting to get support, not solutions. Women can come to understand why men shift the topic to something they did and/or something they know about, rather than asking questions as a woman would (asking questions might suggest the other person know more). Many men relish getting into lively arguments about politics, sports, or a professional issue. Like boys at play, men are establishing their place in the pecking order. They enjoy the competitive process; for example, men like their debate opponents' better afterwards; women tend to like any challenger or debater less afterwards.

If we fully recognize these major differences between men and women and we can understand that the man, trying to be helpful, offers his wife a solution to the problem she is sharing; she gets angry because he seems to be assuming that he could handle the problem better than she could. Besides, his giving advice cut her off from telling all the details and her feelings! He can't understand why she becomes mad at him after he tries to help, then he gets mad at her for being a "typical woman."

This is a serious communication problem. Women start more conversations than men, ask more questions, attempt to put the other person at ease more, are more supportive of the talker, and generally take more responsibility for the overall social situation. These are valuable, commendable skills. Men not only change the topic more but they do 95% of the interrupting of women in mixed company. This is observable chauvinism.

Men and Women Respond Differently To New and Challenging Ideas.

"A woman has the last word in any argument. Anything a man says after that is the beginning of a new argument."

The book *Women's Ways of Knowing* by Belenky, Clinchy, Goldberger & Tarule (1986) describes a feminine learning style that fits well with women's conversational style. Example: When women hear a new or different idea, they set their doubts and disbelief aside and tune in carefully to what the person is saying; they try to see it from the other person's viewpoint. Women try to understand the other person's opinion as completely and deeply as possible; they cognitively "go with them," wanting to hear the person's views and understand why he or she thinks this way. Women seek to make sense of the new idea, to grasp how it can be seen as accurate and useful. This is certainly a "way of knowing" and could be called the "believing approach". It involves empathizing with the speaker to cooperatively assimilate the truth together, i.e. cooperating. Women effectively use this same listening style when someone has a personal problem.

Contrast this with a common male approach: When someone expresses a new idea or one you (a male) don't agree with, you immediately start arguing in your head. You try to stay unbiased and coolly impersonal, if you can, but you question the validity of everything--"How do you know that?" "Is that logical?" "How reliably was that measured?" "Aren't some other experimental approaches or control conditions needed?" "Aren't there exceptions or other explanations or conclusions possible?" "What are this person's motives and biases?"

This is critical thinking; it is the essence of the scientific method; you could call it an adversarial or "doubting approach." You all know this approach; researchers attack each other's conclusions; it is about all you get in school. In academia it is the only respected way of knowing. Men like the intellectual game. It is like arguing--trying to find out who is superior. Women frequently dislike this kind of discourse, believing arguments don't influence anyone's thinking and reduce intimacy. Some careful thought will surely convince you that every person needs to use both "ways of knowing". Both are valuable skills.

Sex In a Committed Relationship

It's a fact that we are marrying later. In 1975, 65% of women had married by age 25 and 93% by their early 30's. In 1990, only 40% of women have married by age 25 and only 82% are married by their early 30's. But we aren't postponing sex until marriage. Between 18 and the middle or late 20's, before marriage we are often involved with a series of sexual partners in more prolonged and "committed" relationships. In their lifetime, 55% of men and 30% of women have had 5 or more sex partners (20% of men and 30% of women have had only one partner). The sexually active singles are not unhappy with their lot, as only one in three would prefer being married. Indeed, as long as there are no children, these serious premarital relationships are something like the early part of a marriage.

Once started, sex is usually frequent during the first few months of a sexual relationship. After the intensely sexual beginning, intercourse gradually declines over the next 2 to 4 years so that at age 25 or 30 the average couple, who have been married 5 years or so, make love maybe twice a week. At 40 it's about 1 1/2 times a week. In a recent survey, 45% of married couples said they had sex "a few times a month" and 35% said "2-3 times a week." Yet, the average frequency of 1 to 3 times per week (for 25 to 59- year-olds) hides big differences among us. For example, about 12% have sex only "a few times a year". Even some young couples have sex only once every 2 or 3 weeks. On the other hand, 7% have sex four or more times a week; rarely is it once or twice a day (Michael, Gagnon, Laumann & Kolata, 1994). Whatever pleases each couple is okay. Quality is what counts, not quantity. However, for a variety of reasons, men seem to want it more than women. About 55% of men think about sex every day; only 20% of women do.

Excluding the extremes, frequency of intercourse tends to roughly reflect how satisfied the partners are with their sex life (Blumstein & Schwartz, 1983). For example, 89% of couples having sex 3 or more times per week are satisfied with their sex life. Among couples who have sex 1 to 4 times a month, only about 53% are satisfied. Don't conclude, however, that the way to achieve a better sex life is to double or triple the frequency. It's more complicated than that. Overall, about 70% of married couples rate their sex life as being okay (meaning almost one third are dissatisfied). If your sex life is very good, regardless of frequency, your marriage is more likely to be close.

Both men and women occasionally have difficulty coming to a climax. Only about 5% to 10% of men but 30% of married women only occasionally or never climax--another 30% of women consistently have orgasms (Michael, Gagnon, Laumann & Kolata, 1994). Women who are very happy with their marriages are much more likely to be orgasmic (but being non-orgasmic doesn't necessarily mean you have a serious, unconscious dissatisfaction with your relationship).

There are remarkable variations in researchers' estimates of how many husbands and wives are unfaithful, ranging from 20% to 70%. Knox (1984) suggested that 50% of men and 20-40% of women have had an affair at some time. A more scientific survey found that 75% of married men and 85% of married women had been faithful (Michael, Gagnon, Laumann & Kolata, 1994), but these surveys include the newly married. In recent years, extramarital sex reportedly occurs about as often among women as men. Working outside the home increases the chances of an affair for women (Levin, 1975); about 50% of these women supposedly have had extramarital sex. Men seek casual sex and have more outside partners; women seek emotional attachment and have fewer outside partners (Blumstein & Schwartz, 1983). Some research suggests, as you would expect, that a poor marriage or unsatisfactory sex is often associated with unfaithfulness (Thompson, 1983). According to Grosskopf (1983), from 50% to 70% of unfaithful women said they did it because they were emotionally and sexually dissatisfied with their husbands (35% had found out *he* had an affair). On the other hand, Blumstein and Schwartz say that many couples who have had an affair are just as happy with their marriages as faithful spouses. They also say that having one affair doesn't necessarily lead to another, and that church goers are just as likely to be unfaithful as non-goers. Unfaithfulness has been discussed above.

Sexual Intercourse: Making Love

Sex, if done well, generates positive feelings towards the partner. "Making love" is usually a natural, emotional experience, a part of a relationship, rarely just a physiologically pleasurable act. We are ordinarily very careful whom we have sex with; it is a consciously planned and orchestrated act. Yet, interestingly enough, human sexual arousal is a primitive physiological response that can't be consciously willed; for example, men can't just will an immediate erection, women can't will lubrication. One needs to generate sexy thoughts or physical stimulation; one needs to be relaxed and "in the mood". Then penises harden and vaginas moisten automatically.

It is tempting to say that making love is just doing what comes naturally, but that isn't at all true either. There are many things about intercourse we don't know automatically. For instance, we don't naturally take lots of time, but good sex can't be rushed. We don't know what feels good to our partner, he/she has to tell us. In the beginning of a relationship, the male doesn't know how to locate a particular woman's clitoris or how she likes it to be stimulated. Females often don't know how to hold and stroke a penis. Both sexes have to learn by being shown or told. Every partner is different and even the same partner has different preferences from time to time, so communication is vital. Furthermore, open communication about our feelings and sexual needs is hampered by emotional hang-ups we have to learn to overcome.

There are also many other learned sexual inhibitions and negative emotions we need to unlearn, e.g. it may be uncomfortable at first, but eventually 90% of married couples have oral-genital sex often or occasionally. We may be embarrassed about moving or thrusting and making noises (expressing our pleasure), but an active, "excited" partner is the sexiest experience we can possibly have. It may be very hard to openly communicate about our bodies and what makes us feel good, but we must if we are going to get maximum pleasure. Sometimes, it is easier and better to show (guide his/her hands) than to try to verbally tell him/her what feels good. Your partner can't read your mind, don't expect it. A section below deals with communication. We may be acutely aware of our ignorance about sex and it may be very difficult to say "I'm ashamed to admit it but I don't know about....", but it is important to be realistic and honest.

It must be realized that both you and your partner bring a long sexual history into even your *first* sexual experience. Histories differ greatly: one partner may have masturbated almost daily since 12 or 13 and had fantasies of having intercourse with thousands of different people; the other partner may have stroked him/herself only a few times ever and had no sexual fantasies. We have all been sexually aroused in our sleep 5 to 7 times every night since childhood; some have enjoyed it, others were mystified and disturbed by their sexual responses during sleep, while some denied or tried to ignore it. Your partners' fantasies of foreplay, of the sex acts involved in intercourse, of what he or she might feel, and of what should be done after intercourse may be radically different from your expectations. Each of us has heard different things about sex from friends, movies, parents, teachers, books, and so on. Males and females may bring different instincts into the sexual act. It is important that every lover be aware of and tolerant of the unique differences his/her partner brings to this vital moment. However, that doesn't mean that sex can't be improved over time, providing you receive good instruction.

Most inexperienced males imagine that really good sex consists of getting the woman partly undressed and then shoving an enormous penis in and out of her vagina until they both explode simultaneously with a fantastic orgasm. For men, the fantasy ends there. What terribly misguided notions we have about good sex.

Few women have the same conception of good sex. Instead, they imagine going out to a romantic setting, having a wonderful time, holding hands, talking, laughing, dancing, etc. Later in the female's fantasy, a nice looking, smooth-talking, confident lover tells her about his feelings for her, their future, her attractiveness, his needs for love, etc. She imagines being held tightly and kissed over and over. Her fantasy may include his slowly and gently touching her breasts and later her sexual parts, eventually undressing her and having intercourse, but this isn't the total focus of her fantasy. After "love making" she imagines being held, comforted, and told that sex has made the closeness and love between them much greater. She wants reassurance that she was an exciting sex partner and that the male wants to do many other things (nonsexual) with her soon.

Early in the love making process, the typical male is worried that he will do something wrong or that she will stop him. He is progressing as rapidly as he can towards intercourse so he won't lose his chance; meanwhile, she is hoping for romantic affection and tries to encourage this by slowing his progress. If she expects and wants to have intercourse, she may realize that time and stroking are needed to start her lubricating. He may have trouble finding her sensitive spot (clitoris) and she hesitates to show him (if she knows). She isn't very turned on by his penis; indeed, she may be scared of touching it or repulsed by it (he thinks it is the most wonderful thing in the world and wishes she would love it as he does). In the end, neither may experience much of what they wanted or imagined it would be like. If they are smart and lucky, both start to realize that this is a complex situation involving actions, emotions, expectations, communication, knowledge, and consideration of others, which will take a long time to truly master.

Good sex involves finding out what the partner wants to happen before, during, and after love making. Then each partner attempts to meet as many of the partner's desires as possible. Compromises will be needed.

There are hundreds of books, some thousands of years old, about improving sex. I will cite several good ones below, but in my opinion the most important secrets are:

1. Love making should focus on loving each other by verbal expression and touching. Consider the orgasm as only the wonderful "climax" of a long love session (if you can afford the time). Certainly give up the foolish notion that both people must come to a climax at the same time (25% of men and 14% of women believe this). A book on sensual massage may give you ideas (Inkeles, 1992).

Note: years later in a relationship, less attention may be given to the expressions of love because the goal of both partners may primarily be physical pleasure. There is nothing wrong with that.

2. The male usually appreciates attention to and stimulation of his penis. Do this often during lovemaking and in other situations as well.

3. After lots of skin contact, most women need to have their clitoris stimulated in order to become aroused and lubricated, and to achieve an orgasm. This is why 20% of women prefer oral sex to produce an orgasm. The clitoris is located about an inch in front of the opening to the vagina. Talk to each other about what the clitoris needs to feel good. After some experience, a vibrator frequently provides the best stimulation to the clitoris.

4. Remember that lovemaking is not a test or contest, not a time to measure or count anything. It's a time for carefree play, a focus on love, and a time to have fun.

In long-term relationships, love, liking, and sex are closely tied together. Throbbing sexual arousal isn't likely to occur if the lovers have been bickering all day (although 25% to 35% of couples "make up" by making love). But good sex increases the love ("makes love") and reduces the tension (McCarthy, 1982). In general, couples who have a friendly relationship also have the best sexual relations (Hatfield, et al, 1982). If sexual intercourse is done with tenderness and enthusiasm, if it occurs in a comfortable setting, if both parties are without guilt and concern about pregnancy, it can be one of life's greatest joys, a wondrous event, a cherished memory, a fantastic way to bond with another human being. While all this is true, there are some couples who love each other deeply and enjoy each other's companionship without having much interest in sex.

Needless to say, if sex is done roughly and selfishly, if one person is deceived or hurt, if it results in an unwanted pregnancy, intercourse can be a horrible experience. Also, like all good experiences, sex can be diminished by expecting too much. Sex with the same person, in time, inevitably loses some of its wild excitement; this should be expected and accepted, not taken as a sign of a loss of love. Intense excitement is replaced by comfort and security. Also, if we get "performance anxiety" and push ourselves to achieve 2 or 3 climaxes or to reach simultaneous orgasms (see Knox, 1984, p. 302), we have to work too hard and set the stage for being disappointed. Once we become a full-time "spectator" observing, coaching, and criticizing our own sexual performance or our partner's, rather than flowing with the feelings, we are in trouble. Worry and anxiety are not a part of good sex.

Books For Improving Sex

There are many good books for learning about sex. For an excellent, up-to-date, informative general text about sex and love, look up Masters, Johnson, and Kolodny (1994). Although somewhat dated, mental health professionals consider Barbach's (1975, 1980, 1982, 1992) books to be the best guides to female sexuality (Santrock, Minett & Campbell, 1994). The therapists also judged Zilbergeld's (1978, 1992) books to be the best guides to male sexuality, especially the more recent publication, which is solid, sensitive, comprehensive, and thoughtful. For an explicit "gourmet guide to lovemaking" it would be hard to beat Comfort's books (1972, 1983, 1991), but expect the pictures to be mildly pornographic.

Other books focus on improving sex. Among the best are Stoppard (1992); Belliveau and Richter (1970), Gray (1995), Heiman, LoPiccolo & LoPiccolo (1976, 1987), Kaplan (1975, 1979, 1987), Kelly (1979), Leiblum and Rosen (1989), McCarthy (1977), McCarthy & McCarthy (1993), Morgenstern (1982), Nowinski (1988), Pearsall (1987), Penney (1981), Pietropinto and Simenauer (1990).

Tips for Improving Your Relationship:

Everything worthwhile takes effort. You need to work on your relationship to keep it functioning. Some of the ways to improve your relationship are as follows:

Stay Active

Staying active doesn't mean you have to be ready to run a marathon, or work barbells every day. It means that you should generally try to maintain your body - going to a dentist, getting checkups, walking a few times a week. Why does this matter?

This isn't about "looking good". Most studies show that looks are pretty unimportant to long-term couples. It's about being a full partner in the relationship. If one person is always too weak to do things, or complains because of aches, or doesn't want to do things because they'd rather watch TV, this really causes stress in a relationship. When one partner is suffering, it causes difficulties for the other. Both partners should do their best to stay healthy for the overall health of the entire relationship.

Share Interests

Most people divorce or break up because they "drift-apart". Look at the activities and interests you currently have - are you doing things together? Look for an activity you both enjoy, or make an effort to learn more about what she does. Find something you both have fun doing together, and look forward to the time you spend with her.

Take A Walk

A lot of being content in a relationship involves being content with yourself - and being happy with how you spend time with your partner. If you're always grousing about not having energy to do things, or are prodding your partner off the couch, it's time for a walk!

Walks let you spend quiet time together, burn calories, and get you out into nature. What could be better?

Turn Off The TV

If your habit is to come home and turn on the TV, try leaving it off for a night. Put on some music, sit and read a picture book together, or play a game. Pass the evening by spending time with each other.

Fun Is Important!

If you survey couples that have stayed together for years and years, and ask them what helped them stay together that long, most will say that they "enjoy" each other! It's human nature; you stay if you're happy. Learn how to make your own relationship fun, so both you and your partner enjoy it for years to come!

A Sense Of Humor

One key trait that researchers find in just about every long- lasting couple is a good sense of humor. If the couple can laugh about things that go wrong, and enjoy life even when it's not perfect, that gives them the resiliency to weather life's ups and downs.

Celebrate Small Victories

Don't leave celebrations for the monumental events. Celebrate when small things happen, and keep that aspect of being special going. It can be a project completed at work, or a task at home finally done - grab some Champagne and spend the time together as a reward.

Get A Gift She Can Use

Getting flowers or candy as a present is an "I remembered" not an "I care" gift. She will appreciate a gift such as a gift certificate for a massage and pedicure because it's something she can use.

Don't Smoke

Researchers have found that not smoking is key to a couple lasting a long time together. Part of what researchers found was that smokers died much earlier, so their ability to have a long relationship was cut short. Also, researchers found that smokers ran into all sorts of health problems, which caused tension and problems in relationships. Smoking also often caused social problems, especially when one partner smoked and the other didn't.

Regardless of how you feel about smoking as a health or individual-choice issue, you should consider that many, many researchers are finding direct correlations between smoking and length of time together.

Show Your Appreciation

Partners do many things for each other each week. Be sure to let your partner know how much you appreciate the things done for you. Making sure that neither of you feels taken for granted is a huge step towards helping the relationship last

Radiate Positive Feelings

You and your partner can help each other through the day by making an effort to be upbeat, smile, laugh, and joke. Coming home to a smiling face and open arms can make a huge difference in someone's day. Coming home with a new joke to tell and a nibble for your partner can cheer up the one who's been waiting.

Be There For Your Partner

It may be a little thing, an after-office get together, or shopping, or something that seems unimportant. However, making the time to be there and spend time with your partner and her friends can be a huge boost to a relationship. It shows in a real, live way that you DO care and want to spend time with her.

It's also an act that ripples outward - now your partner's friends will comment that it was nice for you to show up, reinforcing the act.

Packing For A Trip

When she is packing to go away on a trip, tuck a small present into a corner of the suitcase or bag. It doesn't need to be anything extravagant, a small love note or charm will do. She will be pleasantly surprised when she comes across it in a distant hotel!

Take A Weekend Break

Sometimes you don't realize how much the daily grind of work and chores affects you until you get completely clear of it. Give yourself and your relationship that time to rest, recuperate and regain a sense of balance.

Rent a cabin in the woods, go camping by a lake, or get rooms in a hotel somewhere - even just an hour away. Stay with friends or family, or spend the day walking in the woods. Being free of the chores and drudgery of home can give you the mental sweeping that you need. You need the time to be able to look at each other as playmates and lovers instead of simply chore-partners.

Keep Growing And Learning

For a relationship not to stagnate, the "partners" within it must not stagnate. This may seem pretty straightforward, but a lot of couples learn this the hard way!

Be sure that you are always growing and learning by taking classes, trying new interests, or improving on the ones you do have. You don't have to do something drastic - even small changes can make big differences. If you feel you're in a rut, you'll project that feeling onto the relationship. If, on the other hand, you feel as if you're learning something new and fun, the entire relationship becomes a more fun experience.

CHAPTER 10 - REDUCING THE STRESS IN YOUR LIFE

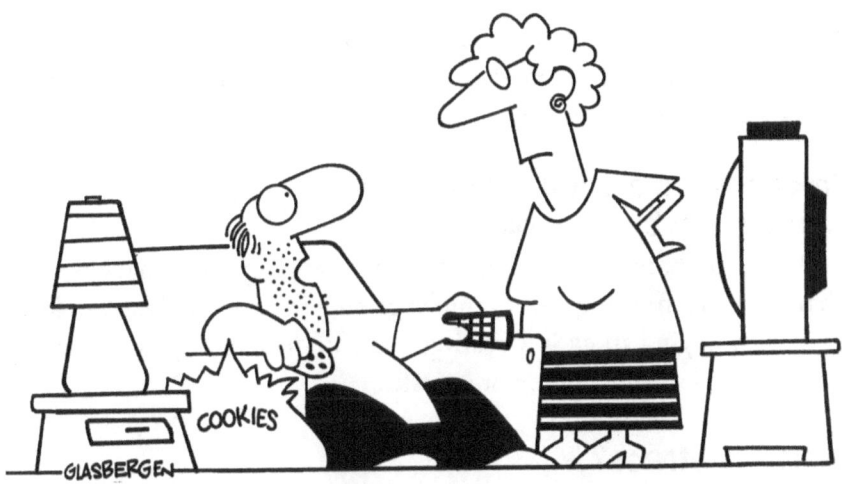

"I am not a lazy bum! I am a potential workaholic
with highly developed stress management skills!"

Common Misconceptions About Stress

We always know when we are under stress.

People often become so accustomed to stress that they become
unaware of it. Many of us suffer the debilitating effects of stress even
though we don't feel tense. Stress can change the way you treat others,
or can damage your body even in the absence of feelings of frustration
or anxiety.

Stress is something that affects only those who have high- pressure lives.

Many ordinary individuals experience the constant stress of worry,
leading unfulfilled lives, or of not being what they would like to be.

The only way to lower stress is to change your surroundings or to take medication.

Changing your outlook on life is the most reliable and effective way of reducing stress. Stress comes from the way we perceive the world, not from the way the world really is.

Stress is caused by events that happen to us.

It is not events in themselves that cause our distress, but rather the views we take of events.

Emotions have a will of their own and cannot be controlled.

We can change our feelings by first changing our behavior or by changing our thinking. For example, getting some work done can keep us from worrying about it. Creating a new understanding of a situation can make it less threatening or stressful.

What is Stress?

The behavioral effects of stress

The behavioral effects of an over-stressed lifestyle are easy to explain. For instance, when under pressure, some people are more likely to drink heavily or smoke as a way of getting immediate chemical relief from stress. Others may have so much work to do that they do not exercise or eat properly. They may cut down on sleep, or may worry so much that they sleep badly. They may get so carried away with work and meeting daily pressures that they do not take time to see the doctor or dentist when they need to. All of these are likely to have a negative effect on health.

The direct physiological effects of excessive stress are more complex. In some areas they are well understood, while in other areas they are still subject to debate and further research.

Stress and heart disease

The linkage between stress and heart disease is well established. If stress is intense, and stress hormones are not 'used up' by physical activity, our raised heart rate and high blood pressure put tension on arteries and cause damage to them. As the body heals this damage, the artery walls scar and thicken, which can reduce the supply of blood and oxygen to the heart.

This is where a fight-or-flight response can become lethal: Stress hormones accelerate the heart to increase the blood supply to muscles; however, blood vessels in the heart may have become so narrow that not enough blood reaches the heart to meet these demands. If you experience this, and you are lucky, you will in turn experience chest pains, will stop doing what you are doing and immediately seek medical help. If you are not lucky, you will suffer a fatal heart attack.

Other effects of stress

Stress has also been found to impair the immune system, which explains why we are more prone to infection (including colds and flu) when we are stressed. It may intensify symptoms in diseases, such as rheumatoid arthritis, that have an auto-immune component. It also seems to affect headaches and irritable bowel syndrome, and there are now suggestions of links between stress and cancer.

Stress is also associated with mental health problems and, in particular, anxiety and depression. Here the relationship is fairly clear: the negative thinking that is associated with stress also contributes to these.

The direct effects of stress in other areas of health are still under debate. In some areas (for example, in the formation of stomach ulcers) diseases traditionally associated with stress are now attributed to other causes.

Regular exercise can reduce your physiological reaction to stress. It also strengthens your heart and increases the blood supply to it, directly affecting your vulnerability to heart disease.

The Causes of Stress in Your Relationships

Taking each other for granted

A common event in a long-term relationship is taking each other for granted. Lovers become less enthralled, less thrilled, less attached, and less interested in each other. When this happens, lovers often feel unloved. That's not necessarily the true situation. The love may have just moved into a new phase. It is amazing how we can feel and show little love when together with a loved one but suddenly become aware of how much we love, need, and want him/her just as soon as he/she leaves for a trip (or shows interest in someone else).

Cathrina Bauby (1973) says that passive withdrawal (non-communication) is a major problem in long-term relationships. Sometimes this "silence" is a result of being taken for granted, and sometimes it is a result of brewing but suppressed anger. It seems like a natural human process to "adapt," i.e. just not notice things that occur over and over, including our spouse regularly doing considerate things for us. We have to remind ourselves to express our appreciation; after several years, there is no strong drive compelling us to show our love. In other relationships, there may be a strong mixture of love and hate. The result may be a hot and cold relationship and, thus, apathy or indifference or "being taken for granted."

Conflicts

No two people want the same thing, not at every choice point. So, there are unavoidable conflicts in all relationships. Of course, both people may hide and deny the conflicts. Sometimes one person is a martyr and will always give in without a whimper (maybe with an ulcer or a heart attack). In other pairs, one person is the dominant one and must win every conflict, even if he/she has to be deceptive or make nasty personal threats. All three are bad approaches to conflict. There are two much better approaches:
1. agreeing to a fair compromise (getting half of what you want) and
2. developing a creative solution in which both people get most of what they want.

Obviously, the latter is ideal but will not always be possible.

Control by others; control of others

Many of us experience strong needs to control others. We want others to see things and do things our way. We want to sell them something. Shostrom (1968) described several types of manipulators:

The dictator: wants to control others by orders, i.e. by virtue of his/her authority, position, status, or rank. Such a person believes he/she knows what is right and what you should do.

The weakling: controls or defies authority by using his/her weakness, sometimes in powerful ways such as "Oh, I forgot," "I didn't understand," "I just can't do it," or "I'm so nervous." This is passive-aggressiveness.

The calculator: sees the world as a contest of wits. He/she is constantly plotting, conning, pressuring, persuading, selling, seducing, or trying to outwit others.

The clinging vine: wants to be cared for, dependent, submissive, and faithful. As a helpless, grateful, "cuddly child", he/she gets others to do a lot for him/her

The bully: uses his/her anger, toughness, viciousness, and threats to intimidate others and get his/her way. The "tough guy" and "the bitch" are common characters.

What can you do about being manipulated?

-First, recognize what is happening.

-Second, stand up for your rights.

What if you are the manipulator?

Controllers or manipulators use five basic methods of persuading or influencing others (Kipnis & Schmidt, 1985):

1. <u>Carefully</u> stating the reasons and logic for changing
2. <u>Assertively</u> reminding and urging someone to change
3. <u>Soliciting</u> others to support your proposals
4. <u>Going</u> over someone's head to get support from "higher ups"
5. <u>Working</u> out a deal so you get part of what you want

Different people use different methods:

1. The "steam rollers" go for broke and aggressively use all the methods—they won't take no for an answer, and may even threaten, shout, and demand,
2. The "rational ones" rely only on hard facts, logical analysis, careful planning, and compromise.
3. The "pleasers" actively persuade others but mostly use flattery, and personal charm and offering "payoffs".
4. The "onlookers" mostly stay out of the controversy.

In a second study, Schmidt and Kipnis (1987) found that the "steam rollers" got the lowest job evaluations, contrary to what is taught by some business schools. Male "steam rollers" were disliked even more than female "steam rollers," contrary to the common notion that pushy women are the most resented. Sexism does occur, however, when you ask, "Who got the best job evaluations?" "Rational" men and "Pleaser" or "Onlooker" women! Conclusion: men's ideas and women's quiet pleasantness are valued, not women's ideas nor men's pleasant passivity.

Note what methods you use to influence people in different situations. Consider the possible advantages of using the rational approach. Nasty aggressive tactics put others down while soft tactics may put you down. Practice relating to others as intelligent, reasonable equals and in a manner whereby both of you can be winners.

Unconscious controlling of others

The manipulations described above involve conscious, overt control (requesting, persuading, buying off, threatening) or conscious-to-the-controller but hidden-to-the-victim control (deception). Beier and Valens (1975) concentrate on a third kind of control--unaware control. Neither controller nor controlee realizes the purpose or goal (like in "games"). The authors say unconscious control is the most common, powerful, and effective control. Many forms of unaware control are learned by young children: cuteness, weakness, illness, fear, anger, sadness, goodness, giving, love, etc. These acts and feelings can all be used to subtly influence others. There is obviously no quick, conscious defense against this control because we don't know what is happening or how. Is there any defense at all? Yes, learn how to detect the subtle control, then extinguish it by preventing the payoffs. It can be done.

Here are the steps, suggested by Beier and Valens, for avoiding "unaware control".

1. Become as unemotional as possible so you can observe the interaction (with the controlling person) as objectively
2. Observe the effects, i.e. note the results of your interactions, and assume that whatever happens (especially repeatedly) was the unconsciously intended outcome.
3. If you got mad or felt guilty, assume that was the other person's unconscious intent. Don't be misled by the person's words or

"logic," don't try to figure out what made you respond the way you did, just note what payoffs the other person's actions and/or feelings led to.

4. Disengage from the relationship--stop responding in your usual, controlled-by-other-person way. Be understanding, not angry. Listen, but don't rescue him/her. Become passive resistant to the controller; then, observe his/her reaction to your non-response.

5. Next is the key step: now, instead of giving the old manipulated response or no response, give a new surprising response that does not go along with what the manipulator expects (and unconsciously wants) but which does not threaten him/her either. Example: suppose a person (child, spouse or boss) gets attention and status by being nasty and yelling. You could start responding differently by simply saying, "It's good to express your feelings." You give no argument, you show no fear of his/her long verbal abuse, you make no concessions, and you don't cater to his/her whims.

6. Give him/her space: just let the other person find a new and better way to interact with you. You should not try to become a controller of the other person and tell him/her what to do; instead, be free to experiment with different styles of interacting with this person.

Driving each other crazy

Sometimes our lover does things that "drive us crazy." We probably don't know how he/she does it, we just know we feel very uncomfortable--angry, put off, used, etc. Bach and Duetsch (1979) suggest these feelings arise because this person sends us a mixed message. On the surface, the person seems to be saying "everything is OK, please don't change" but underneath there is a subtle request for a change. It's upsetting because one can't stay the same and change too. Why are the requests for changes hidden and denied? Because it is scary to be critical, and maybe even aggressive to bluntly ask a partner to change. We are afraid of anger and rejection. Yet, we all have a right to clear information, to our feelings, to some space, and to some power to influence things. In their book, Bach and Duetsch give hundreds of examples of "crazymaking" interactions:

"**Your-wish-is-my-wish**" is when we accommodate every whim of the other person, not out of love but out of fear of having a conflict. Eventually, anyone would want to change this one-sided situation but might, by then, be reluctant to request the change openly.

"**Divining**" is expecting your loved one to know exactly what you want; if he/she doesn't know, you conclude that he/she doesn't love you.

"**Mind-reading**" is believing you know the thoughts and motives of your partner better than she knows herself. This leads to "analysis" which is "let-me-explain-you-to-you", this often drives the other person away since she may need some personal space, not a free, unwanted psychoanalysis.

"**Mind-raping**" is telling the other person what to think and how she should feel, so that she feels confused if her thoughts and feelings differ from your prescriptions.

"**Mind-ripping** " is when you behave as though the other person has asked you to do something, like giving advice to her, except that she hasn't made such a request.

"**Red-cross-nursing**" is creating a need in another person that only you can fill, thus making yourself indispensable. Stern (1988) says neediness and perfectionism force us to try to be indispensable and take on too much.

"**Overloading** " is giving so many facts or orders that the other person can't possibly handle the situation comfortably.

"**Gunny-sacking** " is storing up many, many grievances and then dumping them all of a sudden on the other person. Naturally, these kinds of things can drive the other person crazy.

What can be done about these crazy-making situations? Bach and Deutsch recommend these steps:

1. When you feel you are being driven crazy (stung, confused, manipulated), step back from the situation and try to see what is happening. Tactful, direct requests for change will work much better for you than subtle or deceptive manipulation. Remember that the other person is making you crazy, in this case because

she wants the relationship to continue. Ask yourself: "What changes do they want me to make?"

2. Become aware of the conditions that underlie crazy making--the other person's fear of rejection, feelings of powerlessness, and fear of requesting a change.

3. Do not react with hostility to the crazy making, even if it is very bothersome. The villain is not the other person, it is his/her (or your) inability to be open about requesting the changes needed. Bring these desired changes into the open.

4. Respect the other person's rights and your rights, including the rights to honest information, feelings, space, and some power. Try to lessen the fear.

5. Don't read minds. Earnestly ask for clear information, especially how the other person sees the situation and feels. Share your own views and feelings, and make yourself vulnerable (this reduces the other person's fears). But limit the discussion to the issue at hand. Find out exactly what changes are wanted now by both of you.

6. Check out your assumptions about the other person. This is called "mind reading with permission".

7. Try to arrive at a fair compromise with both of you making some desired changes.

In an unhealthy relationship, one or both of you:

- Try to control or manipulate the other
- Make the other feel bad about her-/him self
- Ridicule or call names
- Dictate how the other dresses
- Do not make time for each other
- Criticize the other's friends
- Are afraid of the other's temper
- Discourage the other from being close with anyone else
- Ignore each other when one is speaking
- Are overly possessive or get jealous about ordinary behavior
- Criticize or support others in criticizing people with your gender, race, ethnicity, sexual orientation, religion, disability, or other personal attribute

- Control the other's money or other resources (e.g., car)
- Harm or threaten to harm children, family, pets, or objects of personal value
- Push, grab, hit, punches or throws objects
- Use physical force or threats to prevent the other from leaving

The Positive Effects of a Loving, Stress-Free Relationship

In a healthy relationship, you:

- Treat each other with respect
- Feel secure and comfortable
- Are not violent with each other
- Can resolve conflicts satisfactorily
- Enjoy the time you spend together
- Support one another
- Take interest in one another's lives: health, family, work, etc.
- Have privacy in the relationship
- Can trust each other
- Are each sexual by choice
- Communicate clearly and openly
- Have letters, phone calls, and e-mail that are your own
- Make healthy decisions about alcohol or other drugs
- Encourage other friendships
- Are honest about your past and present sexual activity if the relationship is intimate
- Know that most people in your life are happy about the relationship
- Have more good times in the relationship than bad

The reduction of stress in your relationship is critical to a healthy sex life and will prolong your life. The next chapter shows you how in a nutshell.

PART 4 –
RULES FOR HEALTHY LIVING

CHAPTER 11 - TIPS FOR A BETTER LIFE

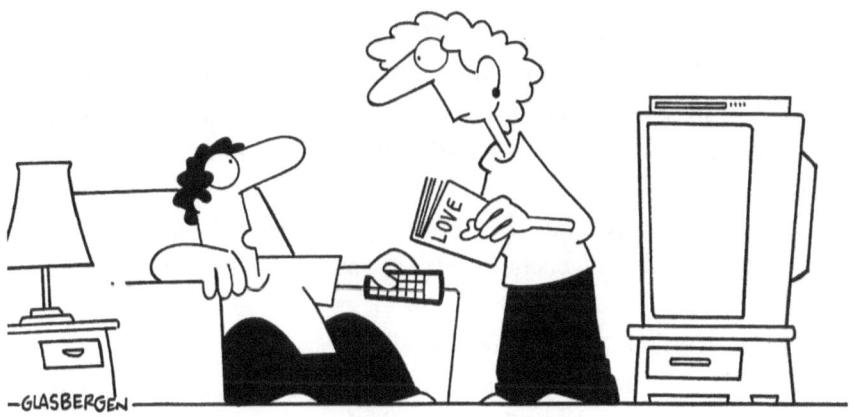

"I do so share my deepest emotions with you!
Hungry and tired are my deepest emotions."

Nutrition Tips

The key to eating for stress reduction is to avoid foods that aggravate our stress response and increase our body's stores of the nutrients we need to handle stresses.

Limit Caffeine and Alcohol.

Caffeine, like adrenaline, is a stimulant. Too much caffeine acts in the same way as too much stress, so caffeine can make stress symptoms worse. Caffeine is found in coffee, chocolate, and many sodas (especially colas).

Alcohol is a depressant and can aggravate stress. All too often, people rely on caffeine to "pick" them up and on alcohol to bring them down. Avoid this stress by restricting your use of both caffeine and alcohol.

Eat Vitamin C-Rich Foods.

Your adrenal glands (which produce adrenaline) use Vitamin C during episodes of physical stress. Illness or injury can deplete Vitamin C. Eating a variety of fresh fruits and vegetables- especially citrus fruits- can help ensure that your body has adequate Vitamin C.

Eat Protein and Complex Carbohydrates.

Your body also uses more protein and complex carbohydrates when under stress. Good sources of protein include peas, beans, fish, poultry, and lean meats. Complex carbohydrates are found in fruits, vegetables, breads, cereals, and pasta.

Note: What you eat can affect how you feel. Follow these tips and you'll improve your health in general, as well as your ability to manage stress.

Tips for Reducing Stress

One of the most effective, long-range reduction of stress is to recognize what causes the buildup of pressure. If you see by your calendar that you are in for a few heavy weeks or too many late nights, block out some relief-valve time. This might be a half- day, whole day or extended weekend. Take yourself out of your normal situation. Place yourself in a situation in which past experience has shown you can forget what is going on. This may mean a day alone at the beach or the mountains, a day with your family or a weekend away with your wife. It's a big help if couples will discuss their future schedules together to identify where the overload problems are and to plan breaks in the routine.

In addition to the count-to-10 pressure reliever, with which most of us are familiar, there are some others:

Staying ahead of your work

This is a good way to relieve the pressure of schedules. By scheduling a completion time 10 percent to 20 percent ahead, you have the peace of knowing there's time to recover if things go wrong.

Doing the hard things first,

Particularly if they have a great deal of emotional content, will relieve the underlying emotions that tend to plague us in different situations.

Getting enough sleep is a must.

Know how long you can get along with a reduced amount of sleep.

Do the difficult tasks in phases.

Often a "first draft" will get you 80 percent of the way along. Time for "topping off" the finished product can be better foreseen, and meeting the deadline seems less of a task.

Have planned recreation and hobbies.

Setting aside time for this activity will help you relax. Find and enjoy different methods of unwinding.

Admitting and verbalizing the causes for your own irritations

Lack of sleep, overworking, too much or whatever else affects you helps keeps others from getting emotional with you and triggering unexpected explosions.

Facing up to the fact that you really can't do all the things you scheduled and that some of them need to be postponed is probably the best relief valve of all. This can be a humbling experience, but the rewards in personal well being are great.

General Tips

Learn To Plan.

Disorganization can breed stress. Having too many projects going simultaneously often leads to confusion, forgetfulness, and the sense that uncompleted projects are hanging over your head. When possible, take on projects one at a time and work on them until completed.

Recognize And Accept Limits.

Most of us set unreasonable goals for ourselves. We can never be perfect, so we often have a sense of failure or inadequacy no matter how well we perform. Set *achievable* goals for yourself.

Learn To Play.

You need occasionally to escape from the pressures of life and have fun. Find pastimes that are absorbing and enjoyable to you no matter what your level of ability is.

Be A Positive Person.

Avoid criticizing others. Learn to praise the things you like in others. Focus upon the good qualities those around you possess. Be sure to give yourself credit and appreciate your own good qualities as well.

Learn To Tolerate And Forgive.

Intolerance of others leads to frustration and anger. An attempt to really understand the way other people feel can make you more accepting of them. Accept and forgive yourself also.

Avoid Unnecessary Competition.

There are many competitive situations in life that we can't avoid. Too much concern with winning in too many areas of life can create excessive tension and anxiety, and make us unnecessarily aggressive.

Get Regular Physical Exercise.

Check with your physician before beginning any exercise program. You will be more likely to stay with an exercise program if you choose one that you really enjoy rather than one that feels like pure hard work and drudgery.

Talk Out Your Troubles.

Find a friend, member of the clergy, faculty member, counselor, or psychotherapist you can be open with. Expressing your "bottled up" tension to a sympathetic ear can be incredibly helpful.

Change Your Thinking.

How we feel emotionally often depends on our outlook or philosophy of life. Changing one's beliefs is a difficult and painstaking process. There is little practical wisdom in the modern world to guide us through our lives. No one has all the answers, but some answers are available.

CHAPTER 12 – RECIPES TO MAKE LIFE EASIER

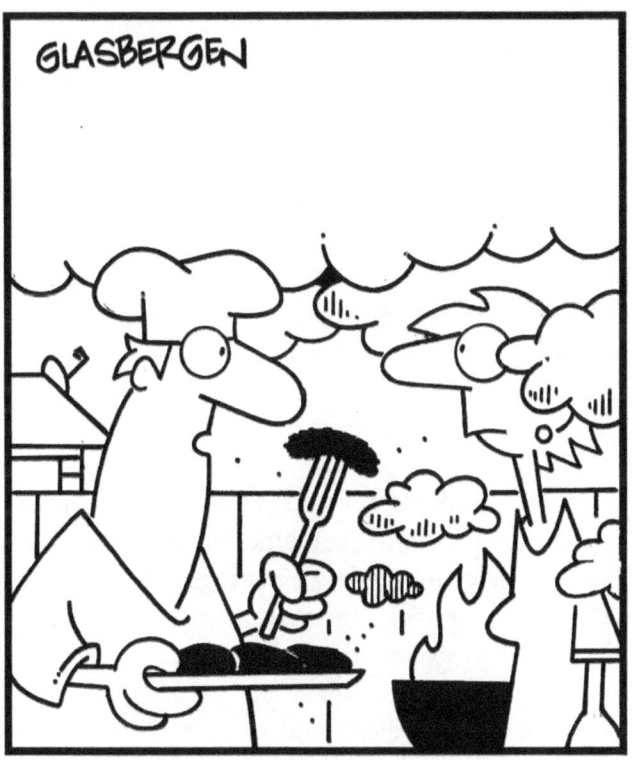

**"Don't worry about burning the calories
— that's already been done!"**

In the cooking domain, it is the barbecue that men have made their own. Can it be that cooking with fire outdoors brings out the primordial feelings of the hunter in men? Whatever the reason, if you are a man that likes to cook there are many recipes that are easy for you to make that can be both delicious and healthy at the same time.

OK so to get you off on the right foot, here are a few simple yet tasty recipes:

BREAKFAST

Oatmeal Muffins

Ingredients:
1 cup low-fat buttermilk
1 cup old-fashioned oatmeal
1 egg
1/4 cup vegetable oil
1 cup whole wheat pastry flour (available in health food stores... it's great for baking)
1/8 cup honey
2 teaspoons baking powder
1/2 teaspoon salt

Directions:

Preheat oven to 425° F degrees. Grease muffin cups or line with paper muffin liners. In a small bowl, combine buttermilk and oats and let soak for 20 minutes. In another bowl, sift together flour, honey, baking powder and salt and set aside. In yet another bowl, beat together the egg and oil then stir in soaked oatmeal mixture.

Make a well in the dry ingredients and add the wet ingredients, mixing until just combined. Spoon batter into prepared muffin cups until cups are 2/3 full and bake in preheated oven for 20 to 25 minutes, until a toothpick inserted into the center of a muffin comes out clean. Makes 1 dozen.

Analysis (Nutritional data per serving)

Calories: 137	Cholesterol: 19mg	Sodium: 154mg
Fiber: 1g	Fat: 6g	Total Carbs: 18g

Baked Eggs with Cheese and Zucchini

Ingredients:

2 teaspoon butter,
2 teaspoon olive oil,
1/2 small onion, chopped
2 - zucchini or yellow squash (12 ounces), thinly sliced
1/2 teaspoon dried basil,
1/2 teaspoon salt,
1/4 teaspoon ground black pepper,
1/3 cup (1 oz) shredded sharp provolone or Swiss cheese,
8 - eggs, large
1 Tablespoon heavy cream or chicken broth,

Directions

Preheat the oven to 350. Heat the butter and oil in a large nonstick skillet over medium heat until the butter has melted. Add the onion, zucchini or squash, basil, teaspoon of the salt, and 1/8 teaspoon of the pepper. Cook, stirring occasionally, until crisp-tender, 5 to 8 minutes. Spread the zucchini mixture over the bottom of 4 individual, shallow baking dishes (or use 1 large baking dish). Sprinkle with 2 tablespoons of the cheese and add the eggs (without breaking the yolks or stirring). Sprinkle with the remaining teaspoon salt, the remaining 1/8 teaspoon pepper, and the remaining 2 tablespoons cheese. Drizzle with the cream or broth. Cover with foil and bake until the whites are set and the yolks begin to thicken, about 15 minutes for individual dishes or 20 minutes for 1 large dish.

Analysis (Nutritional data per serving)

Servings: 4	Calories: 256	Carbs: 6 g
Fiber: 1 g	Cholesterol: 439g	Sodium: 496 mg
Protein: 17 g	Fat: 18	

Apple-Walnut Muffins

Enjoy for breakfast or as a snack.

Ingredients:

1 1/2 cups flour, unbleached or all-purpose
2 teaspoon baking powder,
1 teaspoon baking soda,
1/2 teaspoon cinnamon, ground
1/4 teaspoon salt,
1/2 cup buttermilk,
3 Tablespoon vegetable oil,
1/4 cup brown sugar, packed
1 - egg,
1/2 cup peeled apples,
finely chopped 1/2 cup golden raisins, (optional)

Directions

Preheat the oven to 400° F. Grease a 12-cup muffin pan.

In a medium bowl, combine the flour, baking powder, baking soda, cinnamon, and salt. In a large bowl, stir together the buttermilk, oil, brown sugar, and egg. Stir in the flour mixture until just combined. Do not over mix. Stir in the apples and raisins (if using).

Divide the batter evenly among the prepared muffin cups, filling them about two-thirds full. Bake for 12 to 15 minutes, or until a wooden pick inserted in the center of a muffin comes out clean. Cool on a rack for 5 minutes. Remove to the rack to cool completely.

Analysis (Nutritional data per serving)

Servings: 12	Calories: 122	Protein: 3 g
Carbs:19 g	Cholesterol: 18 g	Sodium: 252 mg
Fat: 4 g		

Banana Pancakes

Ingredients:

1 1/3 cups whole-wheat flour,
1 1/2 teaspoon baking powder,
3/4 cup whole barley, cooked
1/2 cup skim milk,
1/2 cup bananas, mashed
2 - egg whites,
2 Tablespoons maple syrup,
1 Tablespoon canola oil,
2 Tablespoons all-fruit preserves,
2 - bananas, sliced
2 cups orange segments,

Directions:

In a medium bowl, sift together the flour and baking powder. Stir in the barley. In a small bowl, whisk the milk, mashed bananas, egg whites and syrup. Pour into the flour mixture. Stir to combine.

Coat a nonstick skillet with nonstick spray. Heat over medium-high heat. Add half the oil. Spoon in 1/4 cup of the batter for each pancake. Cook until bubbles form on the top. Then flip and cook the other side for another minute. Transfer to a platter and keep warm. Repeat with the remaining oil and batter. Add the preserves to the skillet. Stir to melt. Add the bananas and oranges. Heat for 2 to 3 minutes, occasionally flipping the pieces of fruit with a spatula. Spoon over the pancakes.

Analysis (Nutritional data per serving)

Servings: 4	Calories: 397	Protein: 11 g
Carbs: 83 g	Fiber: 12 g	Cholesterol: 1 g
Sodium: 231 mg	Fat: 5 g	

Cinnamon Coffee Cake

Ingredients:
1 3/4 cups unbleached flour,
1 teaspoon baking powder,
1/2 teaspoon baking soda,
1/2 teaspoon ground cinnamon,
1 cup nonfat sour cream,
3/4 cup sugar,
1/4 cup fat-free egg substitute,
3 Tablespoons canola oil,
1 teaspoon vanilla,

Directions:

Preheat the oven to 350° F. Coat an 8 x 8-inch baking dish with nonstick spray. In a medium bowl, whisk the flour, baking powder, baking soda, and 1/4 teaspoon of the cinnamon.

In a large bowl, combine the sour cream, 2/3 cup of the sugar, the egg substitute, oil, and vanilla. Stir vigorously until well blended. Stir in the flour mixture until thoroughly combined. Pour the batter into the prepared baking dish and spread evenly with a rubber spatula. In a small cup, whisk the remaining 4 teaspoons of sugar and 1/4 teaspoon of cinnamon. Sprinkle the mixture evenly over the batter.

Bake on the center oven rack until a toothpick inserted in the center of the cake comes out clean, 20 to 25 minutes. Cool on a wire rack for 10 to 15 minutes. Cut into pieces and serve warm or at room temperature.

Analysis (Nutritional data per serving)

Servings: 9 slices	Calories: 225	Protein: 5 g
Carbs: 40 g	Fiber: 1 g	Cholesterol: 0 g
Sodium: 162 mg	Fat: 5 g	

Florentine Omelet

Ingredients:
2 cups liquid egg substitute,
1 teaspoon Italian seasoning,
1/4 teaspoon salt,
8 ounces mushrooms, sliced
1 - onion, chopped
1 - red bell pepper, chopped
1 clove garlic, minced
2 ounces spinach leaves, (1 packed cup) chopped
3/4 cup (3 oz) low-fat mozzarella cheese, shredded

Directions:

In a medium bowl, whisk together the egg substitute, Italian seasoning, salt, and 3 tablespoons water. Coat a large nonstick skillet with nonstick spray. Set over medium-high heat. Add the mushrooms, onion, bell pepper, and garlic. Cook, stirring often, for 4 to 5 minutes. Add the spinach. Cook for 1 minute. Transfer to a small bowl and cover. Wipe the skillet with a paper towel. Coat with nonstick spray. Set over medium heat. Pour in half of the egg substitute mixture. Cook for 2 minutes, or until the bottom begins to set. Using a spatula, lift the edges to allow the uncooked mixture to flow to the bottom of the pan. Cook for 2 minutes, or until set. Sprinkle with half of the reserved vegetable mixture and half of the mozzarella. Cover and cook for 2 minutes, or until the cheese melts. Using a spatula, fold the egg mixture in half. Coat the skillet with nonstick spray. Repeat with the remaining egg substitute mixture, vegetable mixture, and mozzarella to cook another omelet.

Analysis (Nutritional data per serving)

Servings: 4   Calories: 158   Protein: 20 g
Carbs: 11 g   Fiber: 2 g   Cholesterol: 11 g
Sodium: 473 mg   Fat: 4

Skillet Scramble with Beef, Eggs, and Greens

Ingredients:

1 large bunch (1 1/4 pounds) Swiss chard, stemmed and chopped
2 Tablespoons olive oil,
1 small onion, chopped
1 clove garlic, minced
12 ounces ground beef chuck,
1/4 teaspoon salt,
1/4 teaspoon ground black pepper,
1/4 teaspoon ground allspice,
3 large eggs, at room temperature
5 drops hot-pepper sauce,
1/4 cup (1 oz) grated Parmesan cheese, or 1/2 cup (2 ounces)
    shredded Swiss cheese

Directions:

Bring a large pot of salted water to a boil. Add the chard and cook just until tender, about 3 minutes. Drain and cool under cold running water. Squeeze dry. Heat the oil in a large skillet over medium heat. Add the onion and cook, stirring occasionally, until lightly browned and soft, 8 to 9 minutes. Stir in the garlic and cook, stirring, for 30 seconds. Add the meat and cook, just until browned, 5 to 6 minutes. Stir in the chard, salt, pepper, and allspice. Cook, stirring frequently, until the meat is no longer pink, 5 to 6 minutes. Reduce the heat to low. In a small bowl, lightly beat the eggs and hot- pepper sauce. Stir into the beef mixture. Cook, stirring, until the eggs are set but still creamy, 4 to 6 minutes. Remove to a platter and sprinkle with the cheese.

Analysis (Nutritional data per serving)

Servings: 4	Calories: 279	Protein: 27 g
Carbs: 7 g	Fiber: 2 g	Cholesterol: 209 g
Sodium: 706 mg	Fat: 17	

Wholesome Oat Muffins

Ingredients:

1 cup & 2 Tablespoons oats,
1 cup buttermilk,
1 cup unbleached all-purpose flour,
1 1/2 teaspoon baking powder,
1/2 teaspoon baking soda,
1/4 teaspoon ground cinnamon,
1/4 teaspoon salt,
1/3 cup vegetable oil,
1 - egg,
1/3 cup brown sugar,, packed
1 teaspoon vanilla extract,

Directions:

Preheat the oven to 425°F. Grease a 12-cup muffin pan. In a small bowl, combine 1 cup of the oats and the

buttermilk. Soak for 30 minutes. In a medium bowl, combine the flour, baking powder, baking soda, cinnamon, and salt. In a large bowl, stir together the oil, egg, brown sugar and vanilla extract until well blended. Stir in the oat mixture. Stir in the flour mixture until just combined. Do not over-mix. Divide the batter evenly among the prepared muffin cups, filling them about two-thirds full. Sprinkle the remaining 2 tablespoons oats over the muffins. Bake for 11 to 15 minutes, or until a wooden pick inserted in the center of a muffin comes out clean. Cool on a rack for 5 minutes. Remove to the rack to cool completely.

Analysis (Nutritional data per serving)

Servings: 12	Calories: 161	Protein: 4 g
Carbs: 21 g	Fiber: 1 g	Cholesterol: 18 g
Sodium: 191 mg	Fat: 7 g	

APPETIZERS

Baked Potato Skins

Ingredients:
1 large russet potato,
2 large sweet potatoes,
1/2 cup (2 oz) Parmesan cheese, grated
1 Tablespoon parsley, chopped
1 teaspoon dried basil leaves,
1/2 teaspoon garlic powder,
1/2 teaspoon salt,
1/2 cup (4 oz) fat-free sour cream,
2 Tablespoons chopped fresh chives or scallion greens,

Directions:

Preheat the oven to 425° F. Line a baking sheet with foil. Pierce the potatoes a few times with a fork. Place on the prepared baking sheet. Bake for 50 to 60 minutes, or until easily pierced with a fork. Remove and allow to cool slightly. Meanwhile, in a small bowl, combine the Parmesan, parsley, basil, garlic powder, and salt. When the potatoes are cool enough to handle, quarter them lengthwise. Scoop out the flesh, leaving a 1/4-inch-thick shell. Reserve the flesh for another use. Cut the strips in half crosswise. You should have 24 wedges. Place on the foil-lined baking sheet. Coat both sides with nonstick spray. Sprinkle with the Parmesan mixture. Bake for 10 to 12 minutes, or until golden brown. To serve, top with dollops of sour cream. Sprinkle with the chives or scallions.

Analysis (Nutritional data per serving)

Servings: 8	Calories: 92	Protein: 5 g
Carbs: 12 g	Fiber: 1 g	Cholesterol: 7 g
Sodium: 373 mg		

Creamy Onion-Pepper Dip

Ingredients:

1 - red onion, chopped
2 teaspoon olive oil,
3/4 cup canned roasted red peppers, chopped
3 ounces fat-free cream cheese,
6 Tablespoons nonfat plain yogurt,
2 Tablespoons fat-free Italian dressing,

Directions:

In a small nonstick skillet over medium-high heat, cook the onion in the oil until very tender, 6 to 8 minutes.

In a food processor, process the onion, peppers, cream cheese, yogurt, and Italian dressing until smooth. Cover and refrigerate for at least 1 hour before serving.

Analysis (Nutritional data per serving)

Servings: 8	Calories: 41	Protein: 2 g
Carbs: 5 g	Fiber: 0 g	Cholesterol: 1 g
Sodium: 187 mg	Fat: 1 g	

Honey-Dijon Chicken Bites

Toss over rice for a tasty meal in no time.

Ingredients:

1/2 cup honey,
2 Tablespoons lemon juice,
1 Tablespoon coarse mustard,
2 Tablespoons Dijon mustard,
2 teaspoon low-sodium soy sauce,
1 pound boneless, skinless chicken breast halves, cut into 1- inch (2.5-cm) pieces
2 Tablespoons fresh parsley, snipped

Directions:

Preheat oven to 375°F.

Combine honey, juice, mustards, and soy sauce. Stir in chicken. Let stand for 10 minutes.

Meanwhile, line a pan with foil. Remove chicken from marinade and place in pan. Bake until chicken is browned and no longer pink in the center, 20 to 25 minutes. Sprinkle with parsley.

Analysis (Nutritional data per serving)

Servings: 4	Calories: 285	Protein: 28 g
Carbs: 38 g	Fiber: 0 g	Cholesterol: 66 g
Sodium: 355 mg		

Italian Salsa and Chips

Making your own chips is an easy way to cut down on fat.

Ingredients:

CHIPS,
1 pkg (10 oz) whole-wheat pitas, 6-inch (15-cm) diameter
1/4 cup (1 oz) Parmesan cheese, grated
1 1/2 t Italian seasoning,

SALSA,
5 - plum tomatoes, chopped
1 small onion, chopped
3/4 cup fresh basil, chopped
3 Tablespoons balsamic or wine vinegar,
2 Tablespoons kalamata olives, chopped
1 Tablespoon olive oil,
2 cloves garlic, chopped
1/4 teaspoon salt,
1/4 teaspoon ground black pepper,

Directions:

To Make the Chips: Preheat the oven to 375°F.
Cover a baking sheet with foil. Cut the pitas into quarters. Separate each wedge into two pieces. Place on the baking sheet. Lightly coat the pitas with nonstick spray. In a small bowl, combine the Parmesan and Italian seasoning. Sprinkle over the pitas. Bake for 8 to 10 minutes, or until golden and crisp. Transfer to a platter or serving basket.

To Make the Salsa: Meanwhile, in a medium bowl, combine the tomatoes, onion, basil, vinegar, olives, oil, garlic, salt, and pepper. Serve with the chips.

Analysis (Nutritional data per serving)

Servings: 6	Calories: 203	Protein: 7 g
Carbs: 32 g	Fiber: 5 g	Cholesterol: 3 g
Sodium: 510 mg	Fat: 6 g	

Pig in a Pinwheel

Ingredients:

1 5-oz can Hormel chunk lean ham, drained
2 8-oz cans crescent-roll dough, reduced-fat refrigerated crescent-roll dough
1/3 cup cream cheese, reduced-fat cream cheese
1/2 cup onion, chopped onion
1 teaspoon oregano, dried oregano

Directions:

Mash the ham, onion, and oregano into the cream cheese. Unroll the dough, which is perforated into 16 triangles. Separate it into eight rectangles instead, then squeeze the central perforations to seal.

Spread an equal amount of the ham-and-cheese mixture over each rectangle. Roll up each rectangle, starting at a short side. Cut each into four slices. Place on a cookie sheet and squash slightly.

Bake at 375ºF for 15 to 20 minutes, until golden.

<u>Analysis (Nutritional data per serving)</u>

Servings: Makes 32 pinwheels
Protein: 2 g   Carbs: 7 g

Calories: 75
Fiber: 0 g

Baked French Fries

Ingredients:
1 Tablespoon olive oil , extra-virgin olive oil
1 1/2 Tablespoons thyme (or rosemary)
1/4 teaspoon black pepper
3 potatoes, baking potatoes

Directions:

Combine olive oil, thyme and black pepper in a large bowl. Cut the potatoes into half-inch wedges and toss them in the oil mixture. Coat a baking pan with nonstick spray and place the potatoes in it in a single layer. Bake for 15 to 20 minutes, at 475°F, turning them once, until they're light brown.

If you like it hot, leave out the pepper and thyme and use 1 teaspoon each of ground cumin, chili powder, paprika, and dried oregano instead. Add 1/4 teaspoon ground red pepper.

For crispier fries, put them under the broiler for a couple of minutes after you bake them - but check on them often, or they'll burn.

Analysis (Nutritional data per serving)

Servings: 3   Calories: 269   Protein: 5 g
Carbs: 52 g   Fiber: 5 g

LUNCH OR DINNER

Confetti Meat Loaf

Brown rice reduces the fat and calories, keeps the meat loaf moist, and gives it a nutty flavor.

Ingredients:

1/2 cup brown rice,
1 Tablespoon olive oil or vegetable oil,
1 small onion, chopped
1 cup red and green bell peppers, chopped
1 pound extra-lean ground beef and/or ground turkey breast,
1 cup chunky salsa,
1/4 cup liquid egg substitute or 1 egg,
3/4 teaspoon salt,
1/2 teaspoon ground black pepper,
1/4-teaspoon celery seeds,

Directions:

Cook rice according to package directions.

Preheat the oven to 350° F. Warm oil in a small skillet over medium heat. Add onion and bell peppers. Cook 5 minutes, or until tender.

In a large bowl, combine meat, salsa, egg substitute or egg, salt, black pepper, and celery seeds. Stir in vegetables and rice. Place mixture in a round baking dish and pat into an oblong loaf. Bake 45 to 50 minutes, or until a thermometer inserted in the center registers 160°F and meat is no longer pink.

Analysis (Nutritional data per serving)

Servings: 6   Calories: 236   Protein: 18 g
Carbs: 19 g   Fiber: 2 g   Cholesterol: 28 g
Sodium: 659 mg   Fat: 10 g

Chili-Spiced Beef Stew

Ingredients:
2 Tablespoons unbleached all-purpose flour,
4 teaspoon chili powder,
1/2 teaspoon salt,
2 pounds lean beef stew meat,
1 Tablespoon olive oil,
2 - onions, sliced
3 cloves garlic, minced
1 teaspoon dried oregano,
2 cups fat-free, no-salt beef broth
2 cans (14 oz) stewed tomatoes,
1 teaspoon sugar,
1/2 teaspoon crushed red-pepper flakes,
2 - potatoes, cubed
4 - carrots, sliced 1/2

Directions:

In a large resealable plastic bag, combine the flour, 1 1/2 teaspoons of the chili powder, and the salt. Add the beef, seal the bag, and toss to coat well. Heat the oil in a large saucepan over medium-high heat. Add the beef and cook, stirring occasionally, for 7 minutes, or until browned. Add the onions, garlic, and oregano. Reduce the heat to medium and cook, stirring often, for 5 minutes. Add the broth, tomatoes, sugar, red-pepper flakes, and the remaining 2 1/2 teaspoons chili powder. Bring to a boil. Reduce the heat to low, cover, and simmer for 2 hours, or until the beef is almost tender, stirring occasionally. Add the potatoes and carrots. Cook, covered, for 30 minutes, or until the vegetables are tender.

Analysis (Nutritional data per serving)

Servings: 8   Calories: 284   Protein: 26 g
Carbs: 23 g   Fiber: 4 g   Cholesterol: 70 g
Sodium: 600 mg   Fat: 10 g

Sloppy Joes

Ingredients:

1/2 teaspoon olive oil,
3/4 cup red onions, chopped
1/2 cup green peppers, chopped
1/2 cup carrots, finely chopped
1/2 cup celery, chopped
1 clove garlic, minced
2 teaspoon dried oregano,
1 pound lean ground beef round,
1/2 cup reduced-sodium tomato sauce,
1/4 cup water,
1 Tablespoon balsamic vinegar,
1 Tablespoon Worcestershire sauce,
2 Tablespoons light brown sugar, packed
1/4 teaspoon ground black pepper,
1/4 teaspoon hot-pepper sauce,
4 - sesame seed buns,

Directions:

Warm the oil in a large nonstick skillet over medium-high heat. Add the onions, green peppers, carrots, celery, garlic, and oregano; cook for 4 or 5 minutes, or until the vegetables are softened. Add the ground beef. Cook, breaking up the meat with a wooden spoon, for 3 minutes, or until no longer pink. Stir in the tomato sauce, water, and vinegar, Worcestershire sauce, brown sugar, black pepper, and hot- pepper sauce. Cook for 3 minutes, or until heated through. Lightly toast the buns. Place 1/2 cup of the mixture on the bottom half of each bun. Top with the other half.

Analysis (Nutritional data per serving)

Protein: 30 g	Calories: 407	Carbs: 40 g
Fiber: 3 g	Cholesterol: 41 g	Sodium: 399 mg
Fat: 14 g		

New York-Style Roast Beef Sandwiches

Ingredients:
1/4 cup buttermilk or fat-free plain yogurt,
2 Tablespoons low-fat mayonnaise,
1/4 cup (1 oz) blue cheese, crumbled
2 Tablespoons fresh chives or scallion greens, chopped
4 small plum tomatoes, halved lengthwise
1 small red onion cut into 4 slices
3/4 pound lean roast beef, cooked, thinly sliced
4 leaves lettuce,
4 - onion sandwich buns, toasted

Directions:

In a small bowl, combine the buttermilk or yogurt, mayonnaise, blue cheese, and chives or scallion greens.

Coat a large nonstick skillet with nonstick spray. Set over medium-high heat until hot. Place the tomatoes and onion in the skillet. Cook for 2 to 3 minutes per side, or until lightly charred.

Layer the roast beef, onion, tomatoes, and lettuce on the bottoms of the buns. Drizzle with the blue cheese dressing. Cover with the bun tops.

Analysis (Nutritional data per serving)

Servings: 4	Calories: 385	Protein: 33 g
Carbs: 34 g	Fiber: 3 g	Cholesterol: 65 g
Sodium: 501 mg	Fat: 13 g	

Smoky Joe's Burger

The usual, with a spicy kick

Ingredients:

1/2 15-oz can barbecue sloppy joe sauce,
1/2 4-oz can(s) sliced or chopped jalapenos, drained
1 3/4 pounds extra-lean ground beef,
1 egg,
1 Tablespoon Worcestershire sauce,
6 hamburger buns,

Directions:

Fire up your grill to medium. Pour 1/4 can of sloppy Joe sauce into a big bowl. Mix in the jalapenos, egg, and Worcestershire sauce. Add the beef and mix some more. Squish the meat into 6 patties, each no more than 3/4 inch thick. Slap them on the grill and close the lid (with the vents open). Grill until they're done the way you like: 5 to 6 minutes per side for medium (160 º F on an instant-read thermometer) or 7 to 8 minutes per side till well-done (170º F). Toast the buns on the grill. Slide in the burgers, cover with the remaining 1/4 can sloppy Joe sauce, and add your favorite fixings.

Analysis (Nutritional data per serving)

Servings: 6	Calories: 384	Protein: 32 g
Carbs: 27 g	Fiber: 2 g	Sodium: 730 mg
Fat: 15 g	Saturated Fat: 6 g	

Caesar Chicken Sandwiches

Ingredients:

4 1/2 Tbsp. flour
3/4 teaspoon ground black pepper
6 boneless, skinless chicken breasts (if the breasts are too big, cut one
    in half)
Cooking spray (I use my own pump filled with oil)
9 Tablespoons lemon juice
6 cloves garlic, minced
6 teaspoons Worcestershire sauce
Dash of Tabasco sauce
3 Tablespoons walnuts, toasted and chopped (optional)
6 teaspoons grated Parmesan cheese
6 whole wheat sandwich rolls, sliced lengthwise
6 Romaine lettuce leaves

Directions:

Combine flour and pepper. Coat chicken with flour mixture (shake off excess. Spray a 10" skillet with cooking spray for 2 seconds; over medium heat, lightly brown chicken on both sides. Combine lemon juice, garlic, Worcestershire and hot pepper sauce; pour over chicken.

Cover; simmer for 15 minutes or until chicken is done. Sprinkle walnuts and cheese over chicken. Arrange lettuce on sandwich rolls; top with chicken. Serve immediately. Serves 6. Per serving:

Analysis (Nutritional data per serving)

Calories: 484	Cholesterol: 101mg	Sodium: 648mg
Total Carbs: 62g	Fiber: 9g	Protein: 40g
Total Fat: 10g		

Baked Garlic Steak Fries

Ingredients:

8 russet potatoes
1/4 cup olive oil
2 teaspoons garlic powder

Directions:

Preheat oven to 400°F. Scrub potatoes well, then cut into steak fry shapes. In a large bowl, toss raw steak fries with olive oil and garlic powder, tossing until well coated. On a cookie sheet, lay flat steak fries (not overlapping) and bake for 15 minutes, turn fries, then finish baking another 15 or so minutes (depending on how thick you cut them).

Serves 6. Per serving:

COOKING HINT: Get your potatoes in the oven BEFORE you start on the sandwiches... they truly don't take long.

Analysis (Nutritional data per serving)

Calories: 162
Fiber: 2g
Total Fat: 9g

Cholesterol: 0mg
Total Carbs: 19g

Sodium: 6mg
Protein: 2g

Delicious Turkey Burgers

Ingredients:

1 pound ground turkey
1 tablespoon garlic powder
1 tablespoon red pepper flakes
1 teaspoon dried minced onion (optional)
1 egg
1/2 cup crushed cheese flavored crackers

Directions:

Preheat a grill for high heat.

In a large bowl, mix together the ground turkey, garlic powder, red pepper flakes, minced onion, egg and crackers using your hands. Form into four fat patties.

Place patties on the grill, and cook for about 5 minutes per side, until well done.

Analysis (Nutritional data per serving)

Calories: 266	Cholesterol: 138mg	Sodium: 182mg
Total Carbs: 7.7g	Fiber: 1g	Protein: 25.5g
Total Fat: 14.4g		

Tasty Tuna Burgers

Ingredients:

1 (6 ounce) can tuna, drained
1 egg
1/2 cup Italian seasoned bread crumbs
1/3 cup minced onion
1/4 cup minced celery
1/4 cup minced red bell pepper
1/4 cup mayonnaise
2 tablespoons chili sauce
1/2 teaspoon dried dill weed
1/4 teaspoon salt
1/8 teaspoon ground black pepper
1 dash hot pepper sauce
1 dash Worcestershire sauce
4 hamburger buns
1 tomato, sliced
4 leaves of lettuce (optional)

Directions:

Combine tuna, egg, bread crumbs, onion, celery, red bell pepper, mayonnaise, chili sauce, dill, salt, pepper, hot pepper sauce and Worcestershire sauce. Mix well. Shape into 4 patties (mixture will be very soft and delicate). Refrigerate for 30 minutes to make the patties easier to handle, if desired. Coat a non-stick skillet with cooking spray; fry tuna patties for about 3 to 4 minutes per side, or until cooked through. These are fragile, so be careful when turning them. Serve on buns with tomatoes and lettuce if desired.

Analysis (Nutritional data per serving)

Calories: 363   Cholesterol: 74mg   Sodium: 918mg
Total Carbs: 37g   Fiber: 2.9g   Protein: 19.1g
Total Fat : 15.3g

Best Burgers Ever

Ingredients:

2 pounds extra-lean ground beef
1 (1-ounce) package dry onion soup mix
1 egg, lightly beaten
2 teaspoons hot pepper sauce
2 teaspoons Worcestershire sauce
1/4 teaspoon ground black pepper
3/4 cup rolled oats

Directions:

Preheat an outdoor grill for medium high heat and lightly oil grate.

In a large bowl, combine the beef, onion soup mix, egg, hot sauce and oats. Shape into 6 patties.

Grill patties over medium high heat for 10 to 20 minutes, or to desired doneness.

Analysis (Nutritional data per serving)

Calories: 324	Cholesterol: 127mg	Sodium: 563mg
Total Carbs: 10.2g	Fiber: 1.4g	Protein: 30.5g
Total Fat: 17.3g		

APPENDIX

Resources:

Nutrition and Dieting

Atkins RC. *Dr Atkins' New Diet Revolution:* New York, NY: Avon Books; 1998.

Sears B, Lawren B. *The Zone: A Dietary Road Map to Lose Weight Permanently, Reset Your Genetic Code, Prevent Disease, Achieve Maximum Physical Performance.* New York, NY: HarperCollins; 1995.

Heller RF, Heller RF. *The Carbohydrate Addict's Diet: The Lifelong Solution to Yo-Yo Dieting.* New York, NY: New American Library; 1993.

Stein K. High-protein, low-carbohydrate diets: do they work? *J Am Diet Assoc.* 2000;100:760-761.

American Heart Association. *Circulation.* 2001; 104:1869-1874.

American Heart Association Statement on High-Protein, Low- Carbohydrate Diet Study. Presented at: Scientific Sessions for the American Heart Association; November 19, 2002; Chicago, Ill.

American Heart Association. High-protein diets: AHA recommendation. Available at: Accessed March 6, 2003.Nagy R. Dr Atkins' diet revolution: a review. *VA Med Mon.* 1974;101 :383-385.

Gleser L, Olkin I. Stochastically dependent effect sizes. In: Cooper J, Hedges L, eds. *The Handbook of Research Synthesis.* New York, NY: Russell Sage Foundation; 1994:339-355.

Hedges L, Olkin I. *Statistical Methods for Meta-analysis.* Vol 1. San Diego, Calif: Academic Press; 1985.

Vessby B, Unsitupa M, Hermansen K, et al. Substituting dietary saturated for monounsaturated fat impairs insulin sensitivity in healthy men and women: the KANWU Study. *Diabetologia.* 2001;44:3 12-3 19

Hockaday TD, Hockaday JM, Mann JI, Turner RC. Prospective comparison of modified fat-high-carbohydrate with standard low- carbohydrate dietary advice in the treatment of diabetes: one year follow-up study. *Br J Nutr.* 1978;39:357-362.

Baron JA, Schori A, Crow B, Carter R, Mann JI. A randomized controlled trial of low carbohydrate and low fat/high fiber diets for weight loss. Am J Public Health. 1986;76:1293-1296.

Kratz M, von Eckardstein A, Fobker M, et al. The impact of dietary fat composition on serum leptin concentrations in healthy nonobese men and women. J Clin Endocrinol Metab. 2002;87:5008-5014.

Saltzman E, Moriguti JC, Das SK, et al. Effects of a cereal rich in soluble fiber on body composition and dietary compliance during consumption of a hypocaloric diet. J Am Coll Nutr. 2001;20:50-57.

Schlundt DG, Hill JO, Pope-Cordle J, Arnold D, Virts KL, Katahn M. Randomized evaluation of a low fat ad libitum carbohydrate diet for weight reduction. Int J Obes Relat Metab Disord. 1993;17:623-629.

Foster GD, Wadden TA, Peterson FJ, Letizia KA, Bartlett SJ, Conill AM. A controlled comparison of three very-low-calorie diets: effects on weight, body composition, and symptoms. Am J Clin Nutr. 1992;55:811-817.

Skov AR, Toubro S, Ronn B, Holm L, Astrup A. Randomized trial on protein vs carbohydrate in ad libitum fat reduced diet for the treatment of obesity. Int J Obes Relat Metab Disord. 1999;23:528- 536.

Skov AR, Toubro S, Bulow J, Krabbe K, Parving HH, Astrup A. Changes in renal function during weight loss induced by high vs low-protein low-fat diets in overweight subjects. Int J Obes Relat Metab Disord. 1999;23:1170-1177.

Heilbronn LK, Noakes M, Clifton PM. The effect of high- and low-glycemic index energy restricted diets on plasma lipid and glucose profiles in type 2 diabetic subjects with varying glycemic control. J Am Coll Nutr. 2002;2 1:120-127.

Helge JW. Prolonged adaptation to fat-rich diet and training: effects on body fat stores and insulin resistance in man. Int J Obes Relat Metab Disord. 2002;26: 1118-1124

Scott CB, Carpenter R, Taylor A, Gordon NF. Effect of macronutrient composition of an energy-restrictive diet on maximal physical performance. Med Sci Sports Exerc. 1992;24:814-818.

Brussaard JH, Katan MB, Groot PH, Havekes LM, Hautvast JG. Serum lipoproteins of healthy persons fed a low-fat diet or a polyunsaturated fat diet for three months: a comparison of two cholesterol-lowering diets. Atherosclerosis. 1 982;42 :205-219.

Wolever TM, Mehling C. High-carbohydrate-low-glycaemic index dietary advice improves glucose disposition index in subjects

Differences Between Men and Women

Bakan, D. 1966. The Duality of Human Existence. Chicago, IL: Rand McNally.

Bem, S.L. 1974. "The Measurement of Psychological Androgyny." Journal of Consulting and Clinical Psychology 42: 115-162.

Buss, D. M. 1995. "Psychological Sex Differences: Origins Through Sexual Selection." American Psychologist 50: 164-168.

Costa, P. T., Terracciano, A. and McCrae, R.R. 2001. "Gender Differences in Personality Traits Across Cultures: Robust and Surprising Findings." Journal of Personality and Social Psychology 81(2): 322-33 1.

Eagly, A. H. 1987. Sex Differences in Social Behavior: A Social- Role Interpretation. Hillsdale, NJ: Erlbaum.

Haas, A. 1979. "Male and Female Spoken Language Differences: Stereotypes and Evidence." Psychological Bulletin 86: 616-626.

Hall, J.A. 1984. Nonverbal Sex Differences: Communication Accuracy and Expressive Style. Baltimore: Johns Hopkins University Press.

Halpern, D.F. 1997. "Sex Differences in Intelligence." American Psychologist 52: 1091-1102.

Hunt, R. R. and Einstein, G. O. 1981. "Relational and Item- Specific Information in Memory." Journal of Verbal Learning and Verbal Behavior 20: 497-5 14.

Kelly, J.R. and Hutson-Comeaux, S.L. 1999. "Gender-Emotion Stereotypes are Context Specific." Sex Roles 40(1/2): 107-120.

Lenney, E., Gold, J. and Browning, C. 1983. "Sex Differences in Self-Confidence: The Influence of Comparison to Others' Ability Level." Sex Roles 9: 925-942. Witkin, H 1979. "Socialization, Culture and Ecology in the Development of Group Sex Differences in Cognitive Style." Human Development 22 (5): 358-372.

Maccoby, E. E. and Jacklin, C. N. 1974. The Psychology of Sex Differences. Stanford: Stanford University Press.

Maheswaran, D. and Meyers-Levy, J. 1990. "The Influence of Message Framing and Issue Involvement." Journal of Marketing Research 27 (August): 361-367.

Mallick, S. K. and McCandless, B. R. 1966. "A Study of the Catharsis of Aggression." Journal of Personality and Social Psychology 4(6): 59 1-596.

McClelland, D. C. 1975. Power: The Inner Experience. New York: Irving.

Meyers-Levy, J. 1988. "Influence of Sex Roles on Judgment." Journal of Consumer Research 14 (March): 522-530.

Meyers-Levy, J. 1989. "Gender Differences in Information Processing: A Selectivity Interpretation." In Cognitive and Affective Responses to Advertising. Editors: Patricia Cafferata and Alice Tybout. Lexington, MA: Lexington, 2 19-260.

Meyers-Levy, J. and Maheswaran, D. 1991. "Exploring Differences in Males' and Females' Processing Strategy." Journal of Consumer Research 18 (June): 63-70.

Money, J. and Ehrhardt, A. A. 1972. Man & Woman, Boy & Girl: The Differentiation and Dimorphism of Gender Identity from Conception to Maturity. Baltimore: Johns Hopkins University Press.

Nash, S. C. 1975. "The Relationship among Sex-Role Stereotyping, Sex-Role Preference, and Sex Difference in Spatial Visualization." Sex Roles 1(1): 15-32.

Sherman, J. A. 1971. On the Psychology of Women: A Survey of Empirical Studies. Springfield, IL: C. C. Thomas.

Schultheiss, O.C. 2001. "Assessment of Implicit Motives with a Research Version of the TAT: Picture Profiles, Gender Differences, and Relations to Other Personality Measures." Journal of Personality Assessment 77(1): 71-86.

Behavior

Bandura, A. (1986). *Social foundations of thought and action: A social-cognitive theory.* Englewood Cliffs, NJ: Prentice-Hall.

Baumeister, R. F., Heatherton, T. F. & Tice, D. M. (1994). *Losing control: How and why people fail at self-regulation.* New York: Academic Press.

Ferster, C. B. & Culbertson, S. A. (1982). *Behavior principles.* Englewood Cliffs, NJ: Prentice-Hall.

Klein, S. B. and Mowrer, R. R. (1989). *Contemporary learning theories.* Hillsdale, NJ: Lawrence Erlbaum Associates.

Kohn, A. (1993). *Punished by reward: The trouble with gold stars, incentive plans, A's, praise, and other bribes.* New York: Houghton Mifflin Co.

Leahey, T. H. and Harris, R. J. (1989). *Human learning.* Englewood Cliffs, NJ: Prentice Hall.

Miller, L. K. (1975, 1980). *Principles of everyday behavior analysis* (2nd ed.). Monterey, CA: Brooks/Cole.

Neubauer, P. B. and Neubauer, A. (1990). *Nature's Thumbprint.* Redding, MA: Addison-Wesley.

O'Connell, V. & O'Connell, A. (1974). *Choice & Change: An introduction to the psychology of growth.* Englewood Cliffs, NJ: Prentice Hall.

Patterson, G. R. (1971). *Families: Application of social learning to family life.* Champaign, IL: Research Press.

Skinner, B. F. (1953). *Science and human behavior.* New York: Macmillan.

Thorndike, E. L. (1932). *The fundamentals of learning.* New York: Teachers College, Columbia University.

Love & Marriage

Beck, A. T. (1988-9). *Love is never enough*. New York: Harper & Row.

Berman, S. (1984). *The six demons of love: Men's fears of intimacy* , New York: McGraw Hill Book Company.

Bessell, H. (1984). *The love test*. New York: Morrow.

Bireda, M. R. (1990). *Love addiction: A guide to emotional independence*. Oakland, CA: New Harbinger Publications.

Blinder, M. (1989). *Choosing lovers*. Lakewood, CO: Glenbridge Publishers.

Borcherdt, B. (1996). *Head over heart in love: 25 guides to rational passion*. Sarasota, FL: Professional Resource Press.

Bradshaw, J. (1992). *Creating love: The next great stage of growth*. New York: Macmillan.

Branden, N. (1981). *The psychology of romantic love*. New York: Bantam Books.

Brehm, S. S. (1985). *Intimate relationships*. New York: Random House, Inc.

Buscaglia, L. (1984). *Loving each other*. New York: Fawcett.

Chopich, E. J. & Paul, M. (1990, 1993). *Healing your aloneness: Finding love and wholeness through your inner child*. San Francisco: Harper & Row.

Cowan, C. & Kinder, M. (1985). *Smart women, foolish choices*. New York: Signet.

Crowell, A. (1995). *I'd rather be married: Finding your future spouse*. Oakland, CA: New Harbinger Press.

Dreyfus, E. A. (1994). *Someone right for you*. TAB Books.DeAngelis, B. (1992). *Are you the one for me* ? New York: Delacorte Press.

Dreyfus, E. A. (1994). *Someone right for you*. TAB Books.

Ellis, A. & Harper, R. A. (1975b). *A guide to successful marriage*. North Hollywood, CA: Wilshire Books.

Emmons, M. L. & Alberti, R. E. (1991). *Accepting each other: Individuality and intimacy in your loving relationship*. San Luis Obispo, CA: Impact Publisher.

Fishman, B. M. (1994). *Resonance: The new chemistry of love: Creating a relationship that gives you the intimacy and independence you've always wanted*. San Francisco: Harper.

Forward, S. & Buck, C. (1991). *Obsessive love: When passion holds you prisoner*. New York: Bantam.

Fromm, E. (1962, 1974). *The art of loving*. New York: Harper & Row.

Giler, J. Z. (1992). *Redefining Mr. Right: A career woman's guide to finding a mate*. Oakland, CA: New Harbinger Press.

Givens, D. (1983). *Love Signals: How to attract a mate*. New York: Pinnacle Books.

Goldstine, D., Larner, K., Zuckerman, S., & Goldstine, H. (1977). *The dance-away lover*. New York: William Morrow & Co.

Gottman, J., Notarius, C., Gonso, J. & Markman, H. (1976). *A couple's guide to communication*. Champaign, IL: Research Press.

Gottman, J. M. (1979). *Marital interactions: Experimental investigations*. New York: Academic Press.

Gray, J. (1993). *Men are from Mars; Women are from Venus*. New York: Harper Collins.

Gray, J. (1994). *What your mother couldn't tell you and your father didn't know: Advanced relationship skills for lasting intimacy*. New York: Harper Collins.

Gray, J. (1995). *Mars and Venus in the bedroom: A guide to lasting romance and passion*. New York: Harper Collins.

Greeson, J. (1994). *Food for love: Healing the food, sex, love & intimacy relationship*. New York: Pocket Books.

Halpern, H. M. (1994). *Finally getting it right: From addictive love to the real thing*. New York: Bantam.

Harlow, H. F. (1973). *Learning to love*. New York: Ballantine.

Hendrick, S. S. & Hendrick, C. (1992). *Liking, loving, and relating* , Pacific Grove, CA: Brooks/Cole Publishing Company.

Hendrix, H. (1988). *Getting the love you want.* New York: Henry Holt.

Hendrix, H. (1990). *Getting the love you want: A guide for couples.* New York: HarperCollins.

Hendrix, H. (Feb., 1991). 10 secrets of a happy marriage. *Family Circle* , 27-30.

Horner, A. (1990). *Being & loving: How to achieve intimacy with another person and retain one's own identity.* Northvale, NJ: Aronson.

Hunt, M. (1975). *The young person's guide to love.* New York: Farrar, Straus, & Giroux, Inc.

Huston, T. L., Surra, C. A., Fitzgerald, N. M., & Cate, R. M. (1981). From courtship to marriage: Mate selection as an interpersonal process.

In S. Duck & R. Gilmour (eds.), *Personal relationships. 2: Developing personal relationships.* New York: Academic Press.

Jampolsky, G. G. (1979). *Love is letting go of fear.* New York: Bantam Book.

Johnson, S. (March, 1994). Love: The immutable longing for contact. *Psychology Today* , *27* , 33-37, 64-66.

Lasswell, M. & Lobsenz, N. (1980). *Styles of loving.* New York: Ballantine Books.

Lauer, J. C. & Lauer, R. (1986). *'Til death do us part.* Binghamton, NY: Haworth Press.

Lederer, W. J. & Jackson, D. D. (1968, 1990). *The mirages of marriage.* New York: W. W. Norton & Company.

Lerner, H. G. (1989). *The dance of intimacy.* New York: Harper & Row.

Mace, D. R. (1958). *Success in marriage.* Nashville, TN: Abington Press.

Mace, D. & Mace, V. (1974). *We can have better marriages if we really want them.* Nashville, Tenn.: Abingdon Press.

Marshall, M. (1984). *The cost of loving: Women and the new fear of intimacy*. New York: Putnam.

Matthews, A. M. (1993). *The engaged woman's survival guide*. New York: Fawcett.

McCary, J. L. (1975). *Freedom and growth in marriage*. New York: John Wiley & Sons.

McKay, M., Fanning, P. & Paleg, K. (1994). *Couple skills*. Oakland, CA: New Harbinger Press.

Napier, A. Y. (1994). *The fragile bond: In search of an equal, intimate, and enduring marriage*. New York: HarperCollins.

Norwood, R. (1985, 1986). *Women who love too much: When you keep wishing and hoping he'll change*. New York: Pocket Books.

Oden, T. C. (1974). *Game free: A guide to the meaning of intimacy*. New York: Harper and Row.

O'Hanlon, B. & Hudson, P. (1995). *Love is a verb: How to stop analyzing your relationship & start making it great!* New York: W. W. Norton.

O'Neill, N. & O'Neill, G. (1973). *Open marriage*. New York: M. Evans.

Osherson, S. (1992). *Wrestling with love*. New York:

Fawcett.Phillips, D. & Judd, R. (1978). *How to fall out of love*. New York: Fawcett.

Phillips, G. & Goodall, L. (1983). *Loving and living*. Englewood Cliffs, NJ: Prentice-Hall.

Pines, A. (1988). *Keeping the spark alive*. New York: St. Martin's Press.

Powell, J. (1974). *The secret of staying in love*. Niles, IL: Argus Communications.

Raphael, S. J. & Abadie, M. J. (1984). *Finding love: Practical advice for men and women*. New York: Arbor House.

Rhodes, S. & Potash, M. S. (1989). *Cold feet: Why men don't commit*. New York: NAL-Dutton.

Rock, M. (1986). *The marriage map*. Atlanta, GA: Peachtree Publishing.

Rogers, C. R. (1972). *Becoming partners: Marriage and its alternatives*. New York: Delacorte Press.

Ruben, H. L. (1986). *Supermarriage: Overcoming predictable crises of married life*. New York: Bantam.

Rubin, L. (1983). *Intimate strangers--men and women together*. New York: Harper Colophon Books.

Rubin, Z. (1973). *Liking and loving: An invitation to social psychology*. New York; Holt, Rinehart & Winston.

Rubinstein, C. & Shaver, P. (1982b). *In search of intimacy*. New York: Random House.

Sangrey, D. (1983). *Wifestyles--Women talk about marriage*. New York:

Sarnoff, I. & Sarnoff, S. (1989). *Love-centered marriage in a self- centered world*. Bristol, PA: Hemisphere Publishing Corp.

Scarf, M. (1987). *Intimate partners: Patterns in love and marriage*. New York: Random House.

Schaef, A. W. (1989). *Escape from intimacy*. San Francisco: Harper & Row.

Schwartz, P. (1994). *Peer marriage: How love between equals really works*. New York: Free Press.

Schwebel, R. (1992). *Who's on top, who's on bottom: How couples can learn to share power*. New York: New market.

Siegelman, E. (1983). *Personal risk: Mastering change in love and work*. New York: Harper & Row.

Shain, M. (1974). *Some men are more perfect than others*. New York: Bantam.

Short, R. (1992). *Sex, love, or infatuation? How can I really know*? Minneapolis, MN: Augsburg Fortress Publisher.

Shostrom, E. & Kavanaugh, J. (1971). *Between man & woman*. New York: Bantam Books.

Sills, J. (1987). *A fine romance: The psychology of successful courtship, making it work for you.* New York: St. Martin.

Sternberg, R. J. (1991). *Love the way you want it.* New York: Bantam Books.

Sternberg, R. J. & Barnes, M. L. (1988). *The psychology of love.* New Haven, CT: Yale University Press.

Suid, R., Bradley, B., Suid, M., & Eastman, J. (1976). *Married, etc.* Reading, MA: Addison-Wesley.

Tennov, R. W. (1978). *Love and limerence.* New York: Stein & Day.

Veroff, J. & Feld, S. (1971). *Marriage and work in America: A study of motives and roles.* New York: Van Nostrand Reinhold.

Viscott, D. (1976, 1990). *How to live with another person.* New York: Pocket Books.

Wallerstein, J. S. & Blakeslee, S. (1995). *The good marriage: How and why love lasts.* Boston: Houghton Mifflin.

Whyte, M. K. (1990). *Dating, mating, and marriage.* Hawthorne, NY: Aldine de Gruyter.

Wilson, A. & Wilson, D. (1976). *Cosmopolitan's living together (married or not) handbook.* New York: Avon.

Zerof, H. G. (1978). *Finding Intimacy. The art of happiness in living together.* New York: Random House.

Zunin, L. & Zunin, N. (1973, 1988). *Contact. The first four minutes.* New York: Ballantine.

Sex and Love

Calderone, M. S. & Johnson, E. W. (1990). *Family book about sexuality.* New York: HarperCollins.

Comfort, A. (1972). *The joy of sex.* New York: Crown Publishers. Comfort, A. (1991). *The new joy of sex.* New York: Crown.

Dodson, B. (1974). *Liberating masturbation.* New York: Bodysex Designs.

Dodson, B. (1987). *Sex for one. The joy of selfloving.* New York: Crown Publishing Group.

Downing, G. (1977). *The massage book.* New York: Random House.

Downing, G. (1992). *The new massage book.* New York: Random House.

Ellis, A. (1974). *Sex without guilt.* North Hollywood, CA: Wilshire Books.Grosskopf, D. (1983). *Sex and the married woman.* New York: Simon & Schuster.

Hajcak, F. & Garwood, P. (1987). *Hidden bedroom partners: Needs and motives that destroy sexual pleasure.* New York: Libra Publishers.

Hite, S. (1977). *The Hite report.* New York: Dell.

Inkeles, G. (1993). *The new sexual massage.* New York: Putnam.

Janus, S. S. & Janus, C. L. (1993). *The Janus report on sexual behavior.* New York: Wiley.

Kaplan, H. S. (1995). *The sexual desire disorders: Dysfunctional regulation of sexual motivation.* New York: Brunner/Mazel.

Kelly, G. (1979). *Good sex: A healthy man's guide to sexual fulfillment.* New York: Harcourt Brace Jovanovich.

Kinsey, A. C., Pomeroy, W. B. & Martin, C. E. (1948). *Sexual behavior in the human male.* Philadelphia: Saunders.

Kinsey, A. C., Pomeroy, W. B., Martin, C. E. & Gebhard, P. H. (1953). *Sexual behavior in the human female.* Philadelphia: Saunders.

Knox, D. (1984). *Human sexuality: The search for understanding.* St. Paul, MN: West Publishing Co.

Laumann, E. O., Gagnon, J. H., Michael, R. T. & Michaels, S. (1994). *The social organization of sexuality.* Chicago: Univ. of Chicago Press.

Lawson, A. (1989). *Adultery: An analysis of love and betrayal.* New York: Basic Books.

Leiblum, S. R. & Rosen, R. C. (1980). *Principles and practice of sex therapy: Update for the 1990's.* New York: Guilford Press.

Levitt, E. E. & Klassen, A. D. (1973). *Public attitudes toward sexual behaviors: The latest investigations of the institute for sex research.* Bloomington, IN: Indiana University Press.

Madaras, L. (1983, 1988a). *What's happening to my body book-- for girls.* New York: New Market Press.

Madaras, L. (1984, 1988b). *What's happening to my body book-- for boys.* New York: New Market Press.

Maier, R. A. (1984). *Human sexuality in perspective.* Chicago: Nelson-Hall.

Masters, W. H. & Johnson, V. E. (1970). *Human sexual inadequacy.* Boston, Mass: Little, Brown and Company.

Masters, W. H., Johnson, V. E. & Kolodny, R. C. (1985, 1995). *Human sexuality.* Boston: Little, Brown and Company.

Masters, W. H., Johnson, V. E. & Kolodny, R. C. (1994). *Heterosexuality.* New York: HarperCollins.

McCarthy, B. (1977). *What you (still) don't know about male sexuality.* New York: Thomas Y. Crowell Company.

McCarthy, B. & McCarthy, E. (1993). *Sexual awareness.* New York: Carrol & Graf.

Meyners, R. & Wooster, C. (1979). *Sexual style.* New York: Harcourt Brace Jovanovich.

Michael, R. T., Gagnon, J. H., Laumann, E. O. & Kolata, G. (1994). *Sex in America.* New York: Little, Brown.

Nowinski, J. (1988). *A lifelong love affair. Keeping sexual desire alive in your relationship.* New York: Norton.

Pearsall, P. (1987). *Super marital sex. Loving for life.* New York: Doubleday.

Penney, A. (1981). *How to make love to a man.* New York: Clarkson Potter.

Reinisch, J. M. (1990). *The Kinsey Institute new report on sex.* New York: St. Martin's Press.

Sheffield, M. (1979). *Where do babies come from*? New York: Alfred A. Knopf.

Sorenson, R. C. (1973). *Adolescent sexuality in contemporary America*. New York: World Publishing Co.

Starr, B. D. & Weiner, M. B. (1982). *The Starr-Weiner report on sex and sexuality in the mature years*. New York: McGraw-Hill.

Stoppard, M. (1992). *The magic of sex*. New York: Dorling Kindersley.

Tannahill, R. (1982). *Sex in history*. New York: Stein & Day. Taylor, G. R. (1954). *Sex in history*. New York: Vanguard Press.

Valois, R. F. & Kannermann, S. K. (1992). *Your sexuality: A self- assessment*. New York: McGraw-Hill.

Weinberg, M. S., Williams, C. J. & Pryor, D. W. (1994). *Dual attraction: Bisexuality in the age of AIDS*. New York: Free Press.

Weinrich, J. D. (1987). *Sexual landscapes: Why we are what we are, why we love whom we love*. New York: Macmillan.

Yaffee, M. & Fenwick, E. (1988). *Sexual happiness: A practical approach*. New York: Henry Holt & Co.

Brooks, G. R. (1995). *The centerfold syndrome: How men can overcome objectification and achieve intimacy with women*. San Francisco: Jossey-Bass.

Communication Problems

Belenky, M. F., Clinchy, B. M., Goldberger, N. R., & Tarule, J. M. (1986). *Women's ways of knowing*. New York: Basic Books.

Brown, P. M. (1995). *The death of intimacy: Barriers to meaningful interpersonal relationships*. New York: Haworth Press.

Gordon, L. H. & Frandsen, J. (1993). *Passage to intimacy*. New York: Simon & Schuster.

Tannen, D. (1986). *That's not what I meant! How conversational style makes or breaks relationships*. New York: Ballantine.

Tannen, D. (1990). *You just don't understand*. New York: William Morrow and Co.

Tannen, D. (1994). *Talking from 9 to 5. How women's and men's conversational styles affect who gets heard, who gets credit, and what gets done at work.* New York: W. Morrow.

Relationships

Aronson, E. (1984). *The social animal.* New York: W. H. Freeman & Co.

Beier, E. G. & Valens, E. G. (1975). *People reading.* New York: Warner Books.

Berne, E. (1964). *Games people play.* New York: Ballantine.

Hamachek, D. (1982). *Encounters with others.* New York: Holt, Rinehart & Winston.

Heider, F. (1958). *The psychology of interpersonal relations.* New York: Wiley.

James, M. & Jongeward, D. (1971). *Born to win. Transactional Analysis with Gestalt experiments.* Reading, Mass: Addison- Wesley Publishing Co.

Johnson, D. (1981). *Reaching out. Interpersonal effectiveness and self-actualization.* Englewood Cliffs, NJ: Prentice-Hall.

Kenny, D. A. & De Paulo, B. M. (1993). Do people know how others view them? An empirical and theoretical account. *Psychological Bulletin , 114 ,* 145-161.

Laing, R. D. (1972). *Knots.* New York: Vintage Books.

Laing, R. D., Phillipson, H. & Lee, A. R. (1972). *Interpersonal Perception.* New York: Perennial.

Latane', B. and Darley, J. (1970). *The unresponsive bystander. Why doesn't he help?* New York: Meredith.

Sears, D. O., Peplau, L. A., Freedman, J. L. and Taylor, S. E. (1988). *Social psychology.* Englewood Cliffs, NJ: Prentice Hall.

Sheriff, M. & Harland, C. (1961). *Social judgment.* New Haven, CT: Yale University Press.

Sue, D., Sue, D. & Sue, S. (1981, 1990). *Understanding abnormal behavior* (3rd Ed.). Boston: Houghton Mifflin Co.

Sullivan, H. S. (1953). *The interpersonal theory of personality.* New York: W. W. Norton.

Men's sexual problems

Carnes, P. (1991). *Don't call it love. Recovery from sexual addiction.* New York: Bantam.

Doyle, J. A. (1989). *The male experience.* Madison, WI: Brown & Benchmark.

Eid, J. F. & Pearce, C. A. (1993). *Making love again. Regaining sexual potency through the new injection treatment.* New York: Brunner-Mazel.

Kaplan, H. (1979). *Disorders of sexual desire.* New York: Brunner/Mazel

Kaplan, H. S. (1975, 1987). *The illustrated manual of sex therapy.* New York: Brunner/Mazel

Kaplan, H. S. (1989). *How to overcome premature ejaculation.* New York: Brunner/Mazel.

Margolies, E. (1994). *Undressing the American male. Men with sexual problems and what you can do to help them.* New York: Dutton.

Morgenstern, M. (1982). *How to make love to a woman.* New York: Crown.

Purvis, K. (1992). *The male sexual machine. An owner's manual.* New York: St. Martin.

Williams, W. (1986). *It's up to you. Self-help for men with erection problems.* New York: Williams & Wilkins.

Williams, W. (1988). *Rekindling desire. Bringing your sexual relationship to life.* Oakland, CA: New Harbinger.

Zilbergeld, B. (1978). *Male sexuality: A guide to sexual fulfillment.* Boston: Little, Brown & Co.

Zilbergeld, B. (1992). *The new male sexuality: The truth about men, sex, and pleasure* New York: Bantam.

Dealing with marital problems

Arond, M. & Pauker, S. (1987). The first year of marriage. New York: Warner Books.

Bach, G. & Wyden, P. (1968, 1976). The intimate enemy. New York: William Morrow and Co.

Barbach, L. & Geisinger, D. (1992). Going the distance. New York: NAL-Dutton.

Barker, R. (1987). The green eyed marriage: Surviving jealous relationships. New York: Free Press.

Broder, M. (1993). The art of staying together. New York: Hyperion.

Brown, E. M. (1991). Patterns of infidelity and their treatment. New York: Brunner-Mazel.

Campbell, S. M. (1984). Beyond the power struggle: Dealing with conflict in love and work. San Luis Obispo, CA: Impact Publishers.

Chesanow, N. & Esersky, G. L. (1988). Please read this for me: How to tell the man you love things you can't put into words. New York: Arbor House.

Dolesh, D. J. & Lehman, S. (1985). Love me, love me not: How to survive infidelity. New York: McGraw-Hill.

Duncan, B. L. & Rock, J. W. (1991). Overcoming relationship impasses: Ways to change when your partner won't help. New York: Plenum Publishing.

Eaker-Weil, B. & Winter, R. (1993). Adultery, the forgivable sin: Healing the inherited patterns of betrayal in your family. New York: Carol Publishing Group.

Fullerton, G. P. (1977). Survival in marriage. Hinsdale, IL: The Dryden Press.

Goldberg, H. (1976). The hazards of being male. New York: Signet.

Goldberg, H. (1980). The new male: From self-destruction to self- care. New York: Signet.

Gottman, J. (1994). Why marriages succeed or fail. New York: Simon & Schuster.

Hanlon, B. & Hudson, P. (1995). Love is a verb. New York: W. W. Norton & Co.

Jones, A. & Schechter, S. (1993). When love goes wrong: What to do when you can't do anything right. New York: HarperPerennial.

Klagsbrun, F. (1985). Married people: staying together in the age of divorce. New York: Bantam Books.

Koch, J. & Koch, L. (1976). The marriage savers. New York: Coward, McCann, and Geohegan.

Lazarus, A. A. (1985). Marital myths: Two dozen mistaken beliefs that can ruin a marriage (or make a bad one worse) San Luis Obispo, CA: Impact Publishers.

Linquist, L. (1989). Secret lovers: Affairs happen...how to cope. New York: Free Press.

Madanes, C. & Madanes, C. (1994). The secret meaning of money. San Francisco: Jossey-Bass.

Markman, H., Stanley, S. & Blumberg, S. L. (1994). Fighting for your marriage: Preventing divorce and preserving a lasting love. San Francisco: Jossey-Bass Publishers.

Maslin, B. (1994). The angry marriage: Overcoming the rage, reclaiming the love. New York: Hyperion.

Matthews, A. M. (1990). Why did I marry you, anyway? A practical guide to the first years of marriage. New York: Pocket Books.

Medved, D. (1990). The case against divorce. New York: Ivy Books.

Notarius, C. & Markman, H. (1993). We can work it out: Making sense of marital conflict. New York: Putnam.

Pines, A. M. (1992b). Romantic jealousy: Understanding and conquering the shadow of love. New York: St. Martin's.

Pittman, F. (1989). Private lies: Infidelity and the betrayal of innocence. New York: W. W. Norton & Co.

Raush, H. L., Barry, W. A., Hertel, R. K. & Swain, M. A. (1974). Communication, conflict and marriage. San Francisco: Jossey Bass.

Reibstein, J. & Richards, M. (1994). Sexual arrangements: Marriage and the temptation of infidelity. New York: Simon & Schuster.

Smith, G. & Phillips, A. (1973). Couple therapy. New York: MacMillan Co.

Strean, H. S. (1985). Resolving marital conflicts: A psychodynamic perspective. New York: Wiley.

Stuart, R. B. & Jacobson, B. (1987). Weight, sex, and marriage. New York: W W Norton.

Viscott, D. (1989). I love you: Let's work it out. New York: Pocket Books.

Weil, B. E. (1994). Adultery: The forgivable sin. Mamaroneck, NY: Hastings House Publishing.

Weiner-Davis, M. (1992). Divorce busting. New York: Simon & Schuster.

Weiss, R. S. (1975). Marital separation. New York: Harper/Basic Books.

Wiseman, J. M. (1990). Mediation therapy: Short-term decision making for couples and families in crisis. New York: Free Press.

Personality types

Adorno, T. W., Frenkel-Brunswick, E., Levinson, D. J. & Sanford, R. N. (1950). *The authoritarian personality.* New York: Harper & Row.

Byrne, D. & Kelley, K. (1981). *An introduction to personality (3rd ed.).* Englewood Cliffs, NJ: Prentice-Hall.

Evatt, C. & Feld, B. (1983). *The givers and the takers.* New York: MacMillan.

Harris, T. A. (1973). *I'm OK-You're OK.* New York: Avon.

Harris, A. B. and Harris, T. A. (1985). *Staying OK.* New York: Harper & Row.

Hirsh, J. and Kummerow, J. (1989). *Life types.* New York: Warner Books.

Jourard, S. M. & Landsman, T. (1980). *Healthy Personality.* New York: MacMillan Co.

Maslow, A. H. (1971). *The farther reaches of human nature*. New York: Viking Press.

Mischel, W. (1981). *Introduction to personality*. New York: Holt, Rinehart, and Winston.

Monte, C. F. (1980). *Beneath the mask* (2nd ed.). New York: Holt, Rinehart and Winston.

Myers, I. B. (1980). *Gifts differing*. Palo Alto, CA: Consulting Psychology Press.

Phares, E. J. (1976). *Locus of control in personality*. Morristown, NJ: General Learning Press.

Ryckman, R. M. (1978). *Theories of personality*. New York: D. Van Nostrand.

Shostrom, E. (1968). *Man, the manipulator: The inner journey from manipulation to actualization*. New York: Bantam Books.

Shostrom, E. L. (1972). *Freedom to be*. New York: Bantam Books.

Shostrom, E. L. (1983). *From manipulator to master*. New York: Bantam Books.

Singer, J. L. (1984). *The human personality*. New York: Harcourt Brace Jovanovich.

Thorn, F. and Pishkin, V. (1974). *The life-style analysis*. Brandon, VT: Clinical Psychology Publishing Co.

Zuckerman, M. (1979). *Sensation seeking: Beyond the optimal level of arousal*. Hillsdale, NJ: Erlbaum.

Understanding Stress & Stress Management

M E Amundson, C A Hart and T A Holmes, 1986, Manual for the Schedule of Recent Experience, University of Washington Press

Csikszentmihalyi, M, 1991, Flow: The Psychology of Optimal Experience, HarperCollins, New York

Martha Davis, 2000, The Relaxation and Stress Reduction Workbook, New Harbinger, Oakland, California, USA

Allen Elkin, 2001, Stress Management for Dummies, Hungry Minds, New York, USA

Goldberger, L, Breznitz, S (Eds), 1993, The Handbook of Stress, Free Press, New York

Don Greene, 2001, Fight Your Fear and Win, Random House, New York

Steven E Hobfoll and Alan Vaux, Social Support: Resources and Context, Handbook of Stress (Eds: Leo Goldberger and Shlomo Breznitz), 1993, The Free Press, Toronto, Canada

Baum, Newman et al.), 1997, Cambridge University Press, Cambridge, UK

Mandler, G., 'Thought, Memory and Learning: Effects of Emotional Stress', The Handbook of Stress, Goldberger, L, Breznitz, S (Eds), 1993, Free Press, New York

Steptoe, A, 1997, Stress and Disease, The Cambridge Handbook of Psychology, Health and Medicine, Cambridge University Press, Cambridge, UK.

Taylor, S.E., 1999, Health Psychology (Fourth Edition), McGraw- Hill, Singapore

Rainer Martens PhD, 1987, Coaches Guide to Sport Psychology, Human Kinetics, Champaign, Illinois.

Food Charts

For detailed nutritional breakdown information on any of the foods in your basic diet you can go on the internet and go to the search page for the USDA nutrient database at: http://www.nal.usda.gov/fnic/foodcomp/search/

INDEX

ABOUT THE AUTHOR

Ira Epstein

Ira is an award winning film and video Director/Editor with an Emmy Award for editing a PBS documentary and 3 Clio Awards for his work directing television commercials. During his 35 year career, he has worked on numerous medical instructional videos and health related programs and was responsible for helping to create the original infomercial for "The Atkins Diet" over 25 years ago. While Ira is not a medical doctor, he started out as a pre-med student at CUNY Brooklyn College where he graduated with a Bachelor of Arts degree with a major in psychology. Ira studied the martial arts for over 40 years, which he began when he was seven years old, under the instruction of a Chinese doctor who not only taught him the fighting arts, but also taught him the healing arts and herbology. This extraordinary education added to his diverse background that gave him his unique perspective on the balance of mind, body and spirit that he now wishes to share with other men. He believes that only through the understanding of eating properly, exercising and changing their attitude and behavior toward their significant others, those men can realize a longer, loving and happier life.

www.ingramcontent.com/pod-product-compliance
Lightning Source LLC
Chambersburg PA
CBHW061303280526
45784CB00002B/873